AGELESS

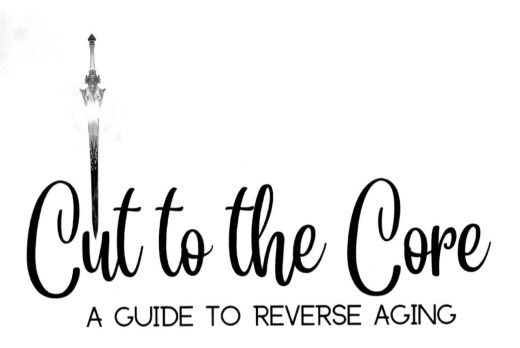

Cut to the Core

A GUIDE TO REVERSE AGING

WENDY JONES

Published by Ageless Wisdom Publishing

wendy@ageless-wisdom.com

www.ageless-wisdom.com

@AgelessWisdom

#AgelessWisdom #CuttotheCore

This book is dedicated to my husband Joseph,

and my children Krista, Robert, Loren, and Logan.

As well as all those who encouraged me to fly toward my dreams.

Let's Soar.

I would like to extend my profound gratitude to Katrena Friel, publisher, editor and believer.

I am grateful to the almighty and to the light, to the God and Goddess within and without who has given us all a precious gift of unconditional love.

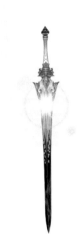

TABLE OF CONTENTS

Part 2 Mind 94

Part 3 Soul 118

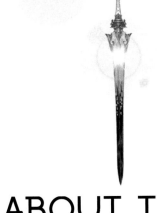

ABOUT THE AUTHOR
Wendy Jones

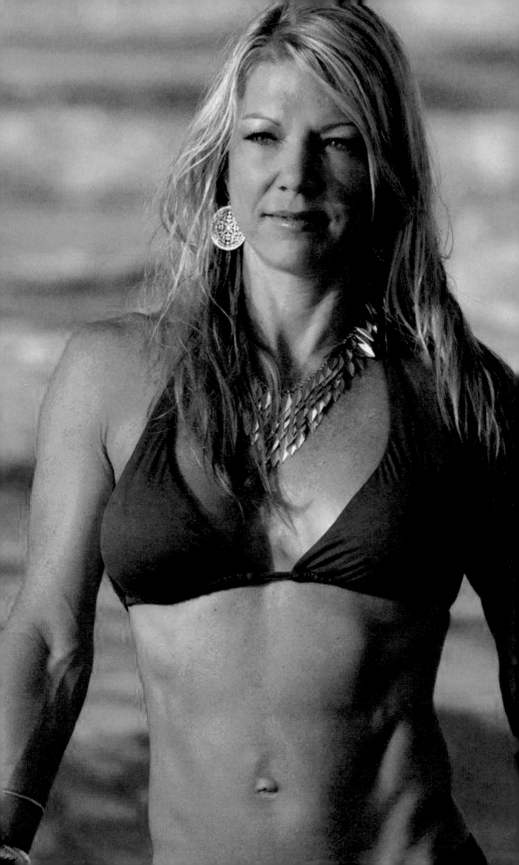

Wendy uses her infectious energy to empower and transform women's lives around the World.

Inspirational and motivational but always approachable, with a matter-of-fact style that is refreshing and down to earth.

She authentically connects with women at a heart and soul level, encouraging them always, with love and compassion.

Influencing her clients to do whatever it takes to become the joyous, powerful, confident woman, that you were always meant to be.

Ageless Wisdom offers clear, timeless insights, bringing you into focus and crystal-clear clarity adding a sense of meaning to your life, motivating you, inspiring you and allowing you to pursue the life of your dreams.

Wendy gives you the magical practical tools and skills to feed your soul while you journey within and bring a newfound richness to the rest of your life.

With every new a-ha moment cracking you open to the infinite possibilities that await you once you learn who you truly are.

Wendy resides in the beautiful, relaxing beach community of North Carolina, USA with her husband and blended family.

Wendy looks forward to walking the path with you, beside you and blessing you in a profound and sacred way.

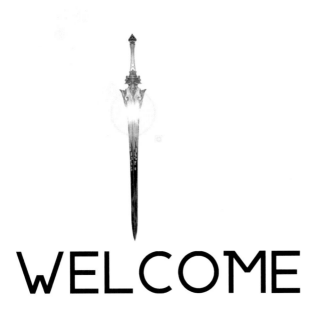

WELCOME

Please come, grab a cup of tea, and snuggle in for a magical read.

My suggestion is to read the book from start to finish to get the lay of the land.

Then come back through the book and take the time to enjoy the exercises, play with the magical tools and do the meditations at your leisure.

We have created a free resources page on the website to download the meditations so you can keep them for your daily ritual and weekly practices.

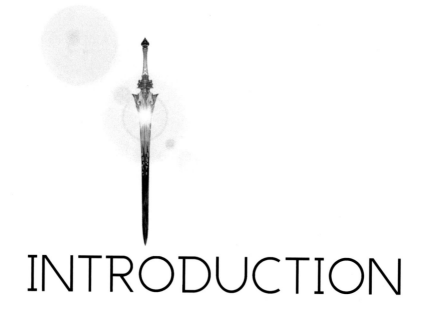

INTRODUCTION

My hope is that you will find this inner journey as life-changing as I have, as you **cut to the core**, and connect with yourself at a deeper, richer level, shedding some light there, and allowing yourself to lighten up and blossom, bearing fruit in your life, for all to see and enjoy.

Imagine all people living life in peace. You may say I'm a dreamer, but I'm not the only one. I hope someday you'll join us and the world will be as one.

John Lennon

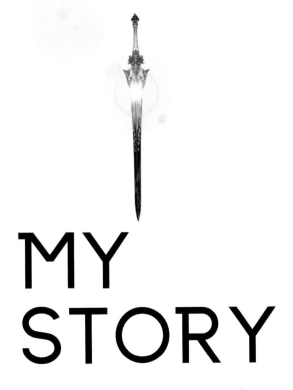

MY STORY

When I sit back and think about my life, I smile.

I smile because all of the beautiful experiences in my life have created who I am today.

I smile, not because all of my life experiences were a walk in the park and easy, but I smile because each one has crafted me into the person I am today.

Everyone who has played a part in my story is of great value to me. I am grateful for every single memory etched in my soul.

I was born under the name of Wendy Lee Davenport, on September 22, 1970, in a small town in the beautiful mountains of upstate New York.

My mother, Charlene was nearly 17 years old. She is the oldest of five children and an Angel on Earth.

Even though she was young, she knew how to show love and we shared a deep bond.

My father was a bit older, perhaps 22 years old and was on active duty in the military, stationed in Germany. He was hardly around.

My mother and I did not have much in the way of monetary means, but we had an instant love that has grounded me and allowed me to build solid roots, seeded in unconditional love. The strength of the love I felt at birth has been the foundation of my life.

There has been a lot of change that has occurred over the course of my life, my parents were not destined to be together, but my life here on earth was. A short couple of years later they were divorced.

The first five years of my life were spent with my mother, grandmother, grandfather, uncles, and aunts.

I loved spending time at my grandmother's house. I would play hopscotch outside, jump on the trampoline, climb trees and walk in the woods to my best friend, Eleanor's house.

I love Eleanor, she and I were inseparable. Every second I could get I would spend with her. That bond was unbreakable, I felt the depths of true friendship, in those early years.

Around that same time, in early 1975, my mother met my father, Rob, the man who has been there for me, all of my years on this earth.

They fell in love, and we moved forty minutes from my hometown, to live with him and start a new life.

They were wed shortly after, I remember being so excited to be adopted and share the same last name.

We were a family!

Even though my life was good, there were times I knew I was adjusting to a new way of life, trying to understand how life was changing yet again. That change continually forced me to come out of my comfort zone.

What I've realized over the years is that change has become one of my main strengths.

Through all the times I might have felt scared or upset, I always had my mother to hold me tight and assure me that everything was going to be all right.

She has always been my rock, my Angel on Earth.

My beautiful Sister Lauren was born in the fall of 1981 and my brother, Jason in the winter of 1985.

They both brought so much joy to my life. They were both so full of life and excitement. I have always felt I would do anything for them, I love them so much.

I remember growing up, feeling how blessed I am to be a part of such a loving family.

Raised in a traditional home, with my mother who was always around, providing love and cooking delicious meals and a father who was a solid provider, protector, and enforcer of rules.

I credit my discipline style to my father, he taught me how to think about things in life, and to be aware of potholes before I stepped into them.

Sometimes that wasn't easy, I was a bit of a rebel as a teenager.

Without their guidance, there is no telling where I would be today.

We lived in a small ski town, that provided my father with a lifestyle that supported our family well. The school I attended consisted of one building from kindergarten to 12th grade, grade school children downstairs, middle, and high school students upstairs.

I kept myself very busy with sports. I thrived on competition and loved soccer and downhill skiing. I remember feeling very proud of my accomplishments during that time.

Even though I was an athlete I still enjoyed the feminine aspects of beauty, makeup, hairspray, and the blow dryer. It was the 80s, big hair was a thing.

I would play cards with my father; my intention was to win his cigarettes. I would put my makeup and blow dryer up as collateral and never failed, I'd lose every time.

My sister, brother and I would dance around the living room, with the music turned way up, singing and laughing, while we could smell fresh cookies baking in the oven.

I cherish those memories with my family.

I moved to Florida, the year I graduated, 16 hours away from home. I was heading south to experience the warmth and to wear a sundress. It was that simple.

I felt the distance of family and missed the closeness of everyone back home.

My siblings sent notes filled with love that brought me back home the following year.

It was 1990, I was 20 years old, and had just moved back to Upstate New York.

As luck would have it, I had the opportunity to move in with my best girlfriend, Eleanor from my younger years.

She and I were having so much fun, reconnecting. Shortly afterwards I met her cousin, John.

He and I started dating and before long we were living together.

At the age of 22, we entered parenthood together.

Robert was born, in January 1993.

As a young mother, I loved the process of being pregnant. It was such an intimate experience.

Being able to feel and see my body change and grow, I felt a deep connection throughout the whole process.

I loved how I was feeling, I felt so much love with Robert, I felt beautiful.

In the spring of 1994, we decided to move south, to the sunny beaches of North Carolina.

As a bonus, my entire immediate family moved to North Carolina around the same time.

Exciting times, in the fall of 1995, we gave birth to Krista. I felt an instant deep love. It is hard to describe the love of a child, it is unique and so special. I was feeling so blessed.

After two pregnancies and nursing for a total of three years, I was a changed woman.

I loved my body, but I wanted to gain back the body I had before my pregnancies.

I started working out at a local gym and spent time learning fitness and exercise. I was lifting weights and cardio to look and feel my best.

I found it to be a great way to rid myself of any added stress. It became my therapy.

I was improving my body on a physical level, but not completely aware of how to love fully, all of me.

I wanted to learn more about the body and decided to continue my education in nursing.

I was accepted into the nursing program at UNCW university in 1998, and worked part-time at a local hospital as a Certified Nursing Assistant Level 2.

With two young children, under the age of four, it took nursing school to another level.

I felt accomplished doing the program but found that nursing was not my intended path after all.

Turns out, I found my calling in beauty.

I enrolled in hair design school shortly afterwards.

I loved being around people and being able to be creative with multi-dimensional color and haircuts.

I loved providing insight, listening, sharing, deep connection, and freedom to transform someone's image.

I have been engaged in the beauty industry for 20 years now, the past 11 years, co-owning a beauty salon with two amazing strong friends, Deborah and Heather. I love them!

We have supported each other through some rough times in our lives, laughed a lot and cried a lot.

We have a strong bond that can't be broken, just like our business name, 3 Strandz.

Braiding 3 strands symbolizes coming together, keeping God and love at the core.

The clear winner for strength is the 3 strand braided rope.

Over the years of working, I have been given the privilege to create some really amazing hair, and image transformations, the trust and respect my clients have shared with me is not something I take for granted.

I honor each and every one of my relationships that have been built around connection, sharing ideas, laughing and crying together.

It's been such a joy to spend time with my clients, each one is uniquely special to me.

I have always loved the beauty industry. In addition to utilizing creative talents, the beauty field also allows me to help and serve others. I am always open to sharing.

Over the next few years, I continued to work out and truly loved fitness. I loved the way my body felt and responded to exercise.

I participated in all types of exercise.

Weights, Yoga, Pilates, Kickboxing, Aerobics, Barre classes, Softball, Volleyball, and Cycling.

I loved challenging my body.

After an injury, that left me facing knee surgery, I was forced to slow down and evaluate life.

During that time, I searched deep within myself.

I was starting to ask myself deep questions about life and my true happiness.

The following year I decided to challenge myself by competing in bodybuilding.

I thought I had a good grip on what it meant to be healthy, I was going to the gym twice a day.

I was doing my cardio, weights and eating my protein.

"Had to get that protein in."

Every morning I had eggs and coffee, a swig of apple cider vinegar, and I was taking my fish oils and protein powder. I was getting in tip-top shape, or so I thought.

I was living a life that felt good but not great.

I was young and unaware of the inner workings of my body.

I was trying, there is so much misinformation out there when it comes to nutrition and how to eat healthy.

It's like throwing a dart in the dark. Lucky if you even come close.

I was listening to friends who were talking about counting their macros and portioning out their food, so they stayed within the proper calorie ranges. That wasn't my style.

I was a bit different. I didn't like the idea of counting calories, instead, I started taking notes on ways to hack the body.

I was very proud and excited when my family, my mother, father and aunt started to follow my healthy food preparation.

They were seeing and feeling results and sharing that information with me.

The decision to compete in bodybuilding required dedication, and a strict, rigorous diet.

I did hours of cardio daily to drop body fat, in preparation for the stage.

I learned the choreography for showcasing my body on stage in front of hundreds of people.

I was disciplined and dedicated to loving my body.

Had I gone to the extreme 1% of those who are daring enough to body build and step on stage?   It was a resounding, hell yeah!

I stepped on stage in 2014, at the age of 44, competing in the women's physique division.

I didn't know much about the sport at the time, but I loved the excitement and challenge. This path required rigorous dedication, training, dieting and cardio.

After four back-to-back competitions, I qualified for a national-level competition. This meant that I was competing for a pro bodybuilding title.

Competitors from all over the world came to compete against one another. I travelled 10 hours to compete and finished 4th place, two spots away from a pro athlete bodybuilder.

Boy, have I learned a lot about nutrition since then.

I have a relationship with my body, 9 years later from stepping on stage that is much more aware. I know now what is truly beneficial and good for my body.

I feel so connected and blessed to have trusted myself and used my body as the barometer to determine what my body is truly calling for.

I was very proud of myself, my dedication had shown me that I am capable of connecting with my body at a very high level.

The love of bodybuilding was something my first husband and I shared throughout our marriage.

He was a strong man in many ways.

Our marriage slowly broke down over the 25 years together, a young love that grew apart over time.

We divorced shortly afterwards.

I am grateful for my friends that supported me through that transition and provided a safe space for me to relax and laugh.

I am grateful for Monica, she has been a wonderful friend who has listened, understood and cried alongside me. I am grateful for my family supporting me, providing a safe place for me, wrapping me in love.

Thank you.

All these major changes in my life have propelled me into self-discovery, self-exploration, and self-love.

I spent years working on finding truths about health and wellness, the truth is, I was seeking happiness.

Showing up for myself, time and time again, seeking out new friendships and exploring new things.

I went to all the local gatherings and learned different perspectives about spirituality, inner beauty, reiki, connection and love.

Finding a beautiful balance, I continued working out daily and refining my thoughts and feelings along the way.

I took an online course that sparked an interest in using my own voice for healing, alongside, kundalini yoga.

I have learned over the years at, 'A Thousand Suns Academy', how to become a living shakti, singing Sanskrit.

I sing Sanskrit, an ancient language of India, that has been around since 1200b.c where it is used as a means of communication and dialogue by the Hindu Celestial Gods.

Energy Medicine Institute in Australia is another beautiful gathering of powerful women that I spend time with monthly, year after year.

Supporting one another along the journey.

I am so grateful for my friend, Dermot, who lives in the UK, 3,812 miles away. His sense of humor is amazing, he kept me laughing, non-stop throughout the year of lockdown, 2020. Friends forever!

All of the courses that I have taken, many books, and friendships have allowed me to evolve and grow on a very deep, spiritual level.

In the spring of 2020, I went to a retreat in Virginia. I met new lifelong friends. Two beautiful, strong women, named Lisa. That December 2020, Lisa J. invited me to Virginia Beach to spend time with her and her husband, Jim and meet some of her friends. I adore them all so much.

I was living life from the book of "YES".

Little did I know, I would meet the love of my life that weekend.

It was on December 14, 2020, that I met Joseph. His humour and the way he showed up in the world made it very comfortable for me to be around him, not to mention he is easy on the eyes.

We became best friends instantly and after six months we started dating.

November 11th, 2022, we married in Vegas.

I gained two adult children, Loren, and Logan that day. We are a beautiful, blended family.

The love that Joseph and I share is unlike any love I have experienced before. I loved myself fiercely first and then showed up, ready to share love.

He is my greatest cheerleader and supporter.

He understands me and loves me for all of me. The perfect and the imperfect.

We share the love of health and wellness.

We share the love of Mind, Body, and Soul.

We are LOVE.

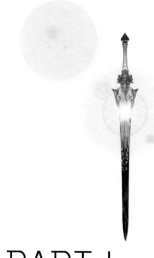

PART I

Body

Seed 1

Knowing who you are

Have you ever just sat for a moment and thought, am I thriving or am I just surviving?

Do I have a deep understanding and connection with my body?

Do I know why I am acting the way I am?

I can go on and on, but most of us seem to be missing a genuine connection with our body. We have somehow become disconnected from ourselves.

Did you know that we are made of energy?

Yes, each of us are made up of energy and our vibration carries information.

These energy fields operate on both subtle and physical planes, as do energy bodies and channels. But fields present mysterious phenomena as well.

Albert Einstein believed that the universe is composed of interconnected force fields. Because of these fields, reality is both local (here and now) and non-local (occurring elsewhere and at other times).

This means that everything across time and space is interconnected.

All fields interact, creating both positive and negative effects on us. The difference between physical and subtle fields is the speed of information and vibration involved.

The physical and subtle fields can actually be looked at as the same fields, flowing into one another.

Fields exist everywhere.

We each produce countless energy fields and interact with endless numbers of external fields. Both subtle and measurable fields emanate from every cell, organ, and organ system as well as from the entire body.

The same thing is true in relation to all living beings on this planet. The earth and other planetary objects emit fields as well.

We also create fields by manufacturing technological products and cell phones.

We are made of innumerable fields, all of which interact to direct, shape, and form our lives.

The physical fields in nature include sound and electromagnetic spectrum. The chief field that generates life is the electromagnetic spectrum, the other is sound.

Each part of the electromagnetic spectrum manifests as radiation that vibrates at a specific rate and is called electromagnetic radiation.

Our bodies require a specific amount of each part of this spectrum for optimal mental, emotional, and physical health.

We can become imbalanced or ill if exposed to too much or too little.

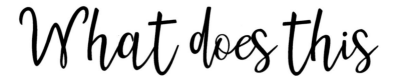

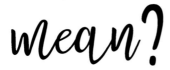

This means you are made of light!

Electromagnetic radiation is described as a stream of photons, the wave particles that are the basis of light.

Sound waves are the other major types of measurable waves. It is important to know that sound waves run at specific vibrations and penetrate all of existence. We can hear some sounds, but not all. This does not however mean that it does not affect us.

Singing, words and language are some examples of sound we hear. The sounds we may not be aware of are our own thoughts or the thoughts of others, both positive and negative. We can chant or sing within as well and receive the magic of sound.

Another important component of the body is the existence of the aura that surrounds the entire body. It acts like a magnetic field of energy that picks up on emotions, health, and psychic circumstances around you.

Your aura can experience stress as you exchange energies with those around you.

It is valuable to pay attention to your inner dialogue, thoughts, and feelings as often as you can and try to surround yourself with positive-minded people.

If you are feeling stressed, irritated, tired, impatient, anxious or develop a negative outlook towards the world, it is important to clean your auric field from time to time.

Ways to clean your auric field include such things as taking a cleansing bath or shower.

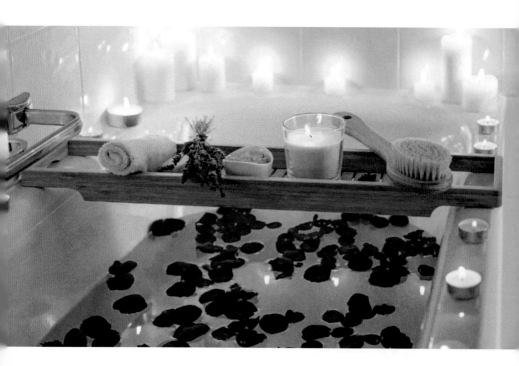

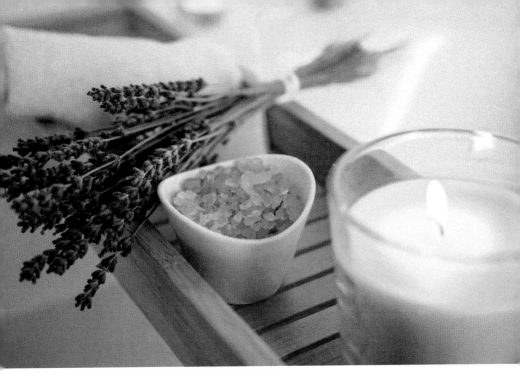

Aura cleansing is a ritualistic bathing process where you make use of salts, essential oils, and sacred herbs to clean your energy field.

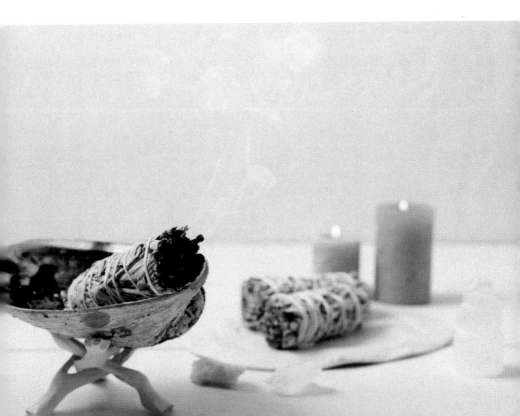

Fill the bathtub, add rose essential oil and a cup of Himalayan Sea Salt. You can add sandalwood and sage to enhance the cleansing effects.

Visualise, divine energy flowing through you, and imagine a white light surrounding you. Take a few deep relaxing breaths and sigh it out.

If you are taking a shower, visualise your aura getting repaired and healed as the water washes over you and starts going down the drain. Bringing in the white, divine energy and allowing it to wash over you and within.

Smudging is one of the oldest aura cleansing practices, using dried white sage or Palo Santo. You burn the sacred herbs by using the smoke coming out of it to cleanse your aura.

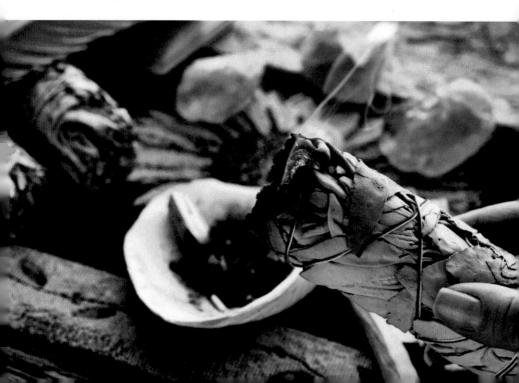

To do this, light the herb and pass the smoke gently over each and every part of your body.

Aura combing is another powerful method that can be done through visualisation.

Start at the top of your head and comb the space around you and go all the way down to your toes. Constantly visualise your aura being cleaned. Follow by washing your hands to clean negative energy.

Chanting mantras and positive affirmations is another effective method of aura cleansing.

Sit and visualise yourself surrounded with a white light.

Close your eyes and start chanting I am beautiful, I am bountiful, I am blissful.

Repeat this or another mantra or positive affirmation you are drawn to. Repeat it as many times as you like until you feel the vibration throughout your body.

Do this daily to strengthen your energy field.

Who am I?

This question can sometimes cause us feelings of anxiety. We may feel lonely and separate. A false belief that only causes us more unfavourable feelings.

The irony is that the more you seek to identify who you are, the more fragile you are likely to feel about yourself.

The better question to ask ourselves is

How would I like to engage life?

Our identity should be seen as an ongoing process. Embracing a flowing sense of self, perpetually reframing, rethinking, reorganizing, and reconsidering ourselves.

Witnessing our thoughts, not reacting out of old habits, and becoming present allows us to better craft our lives.

The identity we seek fires the wave of life, enriched by the flow.

To seek a deeper sense of self is to become intimately aware of your thoughts, feelings, hopes and fears. The key is to be flexible when engaging with yourself, rather than being rigid and hard on yourself.

The universe exists in a state of flowing potential, and you are indeed part of the universe. The goal is to access that potential, keeping the parts of our identity that continue to serve us well and shed the old, habitual pieces that constrain you.

This allows you to find balance between extremes and commit to your personal evolution.

Who am I in this human body?

From the outside, the human body can be divided into several main structures.

The head houses the brain which controls the body.

The neck and trunk houses many of the important systems that keep the body healthy and alive.

The arms and legs help the body to move about and function in the world.

There are five main senses that the body uses to convey information about the outside world to the brain. These senses include sight, hearing, smell, taste, and touch.

The body consists of several organ systems. Each system is made up of organs and other body structures that work together to perform a specific function. Most scientists divide the body into 11 systems.

The skeletal system is made of bones, tendons, and ligaments. It supports the overall structure of the body and protects the organs.

The muscular system works closely with the skeletal system. Muscles help the body to move and interact with the world.

The cardiovascular/circulatory system helps deliver nutrients throughout the body. It consists of the heart, blood vessels and blood.

The digestive system helps to convert food into nutrients and energy for the body. Some of the organs included in this system are the liver, pancreas, stomach, small intestine, and large intestine.

The nervous system helps the body to communicate and allows the brain to control various functions of the body. It includes the spinal cord, brain, and a large network of nerves.

The respiratory system brings oxygen into the body through the lungs and windpipe. It also removes carbon dioxide from the body.

The endocrine system produces hormones that help regulate the other systems in the body. It includes the thyroid, pancreas, adrenal glands, pituitary and more.

The urinary system uses the kidneys to filter blood and eliminate waste. It includes the bladder, kidneys, and urethra.

The immune/lymphatic system work together to protect the body from disease.

The reproductive system includes the sex organs that enable people to have babies. This system is different for males and females.

The integumentary system helps protect the body from the outside world. It includes the hair, skin, and nails.

The physical substance of the body is composed of living cells, and extracellular materials and organized into tissues, organs and systems all working together.

There are all different types of cells in the human body, and when a lot of similar cells work together to perform a function, they make up tissue.

There are four main types of tissue in the human body including connective tissue, muscle tissue, nervous tissue, and epithelial tissue.

Organs are somewhat independent parts of the body and carry out special functions. They are made up of tissues. Some examples of organs include the heart, eyes, lungs, liver, and stomach.

Here are some fun and interesting facts about the body.

Humans are born with 270 bones. Several of these bones fuse together by adulthood making a total of 206 bones in the adult human body.

The average human heart beats around 100,000 times per day.

Fingernails grow much faster than toenails. They are both made of a protein called keratin.

The largest of the human internal organs is the small intestine.

The left lung is typically around 10% smaller than the right lung. This is to make room for the heart.

The human body is made up of around 100 trillion cells.

The human body is made up of four elements, oxygen, carbon, hydrogen, and nitrogen.

Our body is intricate and amazing in its simplicity, with the complex interconnected systems to keep us alive, they all depend on a handful of elements.

When you think about how complex the human body is, that is sort of magical.

Looking at yourself and feeling connected to yourself is so important as it shows how much you value yourself.

If on the other hand, you feel disconnected from yourself, you lose sight of who you really are. You could lose yourself altogether if you are not careful.

When this happens, this often stems from the fear of feeling everything in life is too much to handle, feeling afraid or there's a lack of meaning in your life because you cannot seem to connect with others.

I give you permission to let yourself feel. This may seem like an unnecessary thing to do, but it is so important.

This release will help you stop running away from what you feel is uncomfortable and confront it head-on with compassion for yourself.

Look in the mirror, stare into your eyes and smile.

Date yourself, you will be surprised to find new things out about yourself and how to connect with yourself again.

Make it a weekly thing to buy yourself a bouquet of flowers!

Another great way to spend quality time with yourself is to become creative. Finding your artistic side reconnects you to yourself.

Art allows you to express the things you cannot find words for, which makes it the perfect outlet for all your repressed emotions.

You will feel much lighter by pouring what you feel into your art.

Music, theatre, dance, creative writing and other participatory arts improve your quality of life and well-being, better cognitive function, memory and self-esteem, help reduce stress and reverse ageing.

Cooking is another art form, every meal is a unique manifestation of your authentic voice.

Be free in your cooking style and don't sweat it, there is no wrong or right, only infinite possibilities to embrace and explore.

Allow your love and good intentions to permeate your kitchen creations.

You might be amazed at how impactful your emotional state can be on the finished product.

The more loving you prepare food for others, the more the food fairies will smile down upon you and the tastier it will be.

There is an ancient story from yogic lore about a devotee who prepared the same food for his master day after day, month after month, year after year.

Finally, the servant couldn't stand it any longer and asked his master "How can you stand eating the same food day after day, year after year?

Aren't you tired of eating the same thing?"

To this the master replied, "You have misunderstood. My food is never the same. It is unique and different each and every moment."

The preparation and sharing of food is much like performance art.

Make sure you have plenty of fresh herbs, fruits and flowers to garnish dishes in their natural beauty.

Don't your creations deserve it? Think you are not an artist? Of course, you are! Everyone has something special to offer.

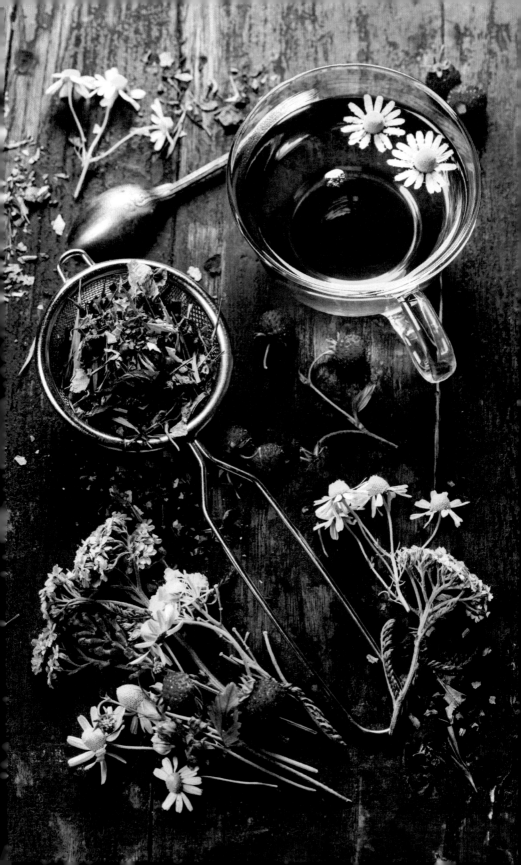

Reflect on how you feel and what makes you happy and what makes you feel alive.

Make a list of wishes and goals, make that bucket list and start planning and dreaming.

With every goal you accomplish, you realize that you get the feeling of being connected to yourself again.

I have found in my life that the simple things really are so important.

I've realized that there is so much to feel alive for, whether it is your loved ones or the beauty of nature itself.

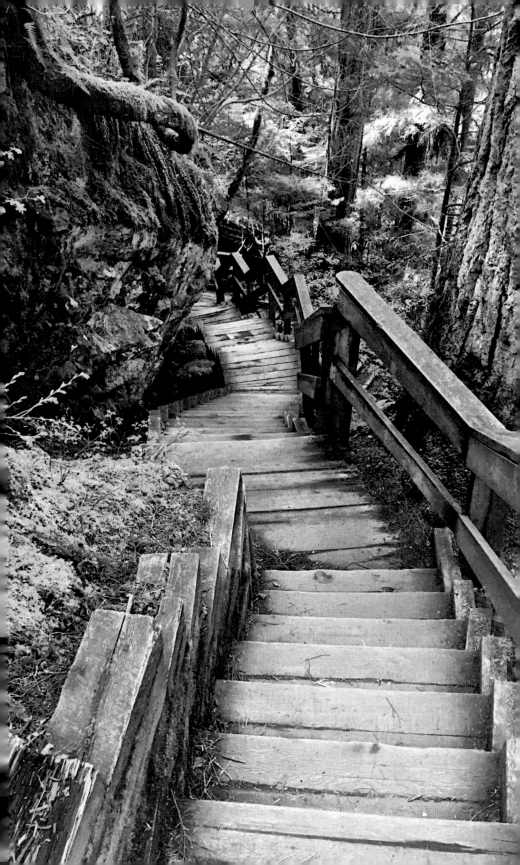

Do things that you love doing, nothing makes you feel more alive than spending time on your passion, such as watching your favorite movie or reading a book you enjoy.

Exercise is also a rich way to connect to the body, since the mind is connected to the body, it is a great way to listen to your body and pay attention to what your body needs and what makes it feel good.

Regular exercise strengthens and conditions the body's cardiovascular network and stimulates blood circulation, helping the body oxygenate and purify itself, adding years to your life.

Going for a walk, swimming, running, jump rope, biking, lifting weights or playing with your animals, all of which will lighten your mood and make you feel more connected to life and to the beauty of who you truly are.

Carve out some time each and every day to enjoy the silence. It is one of the most underrated forms to gain inner peace. We tend to spend so much time on the move and do not allow ourselves a few minutes of silence. You will find that you will be able to connect with yourself and others much better. Life becomes richer and more fulfilling.

Explaining about the Body itself

Do you really know the workings of the body?

Did you know that the human body possesses an enormous, persistent, and astonishing ability to heal itself?

If we deprive our bodies of basic requirements or we are unaware of what truly will keep us healthy over time, we run the risk of becoming unwell.

The most fundamental unit of the human body is the cell, every second that we are alive, the cells in your body are working endlessly to keep you in a state of balance.

Each cell is a living unit that is constantly monitoring and adjusting its own processes, working to restore itself according to the DNA code it was created with, and to maintain balance within each cell.

Cells have the ability to heal themselves, and also to make new cells that replace those that have been permanently damaged or destroyed.

When you cut yourself, for example the blood vessels at the site contract and slow down the bleeding.

The blood plates that come into contact with air, begin to form a blood clot where the injury occurred.

White blood cells will accumulate at the spot to destroy and digest dead cells by secreting special enzymes stored in small packets in the cells, called lysosomes. This way the dead cell debris is removed, and space has been made for the new cell to occupy the space.

The process of new cell formation begins. The healing process is not just for injuries, it also takes care of normal, everyday wear and tear.

Damaged or dead cells are replaced in great numbers every day throughout our entire body including the blood, mouth, and intestines.

The body is endlessly working to repair and regenerate itself. This happens to a great extent when you are sleeping.

If you happen to have a dream that is unfavourable, just know that the body is in the process of healing. The body is letting go and releasing. This perspective allows you to look differently at dreams and the positive connection of healing for the body. This healing reduces stress and helps elevate your mood and appearance.

It is so important to get a good night's sleep. The body requires this time to strengthen and repair the immune system.

I suggest trying to go to sleep at the same time every night, every person is different but typically between 6-8 hours is the average. The goal is for you to wake feeling refreshed and vibrant.

Another way to improve your body's self-healing is by eating a healthy, nutrient-rich diet.

It is important to minimize the consumption of processed foods, as well as artificial food additives, preservatives, natural flavors, acids etc.

A diet rich in vegetables, fruits and low in fats and oils is best.

Personal hygiene is very important for maintaining a healthy body and overall heath.

Spend some quality time on yourself.

Self-soothing touch and massage are very therapeutic.

Start by placing your right hand on the center of your stomach, over your belly button, and softly begin a circular motion in a clockwise direction. Continue doing this for as long as you feel called and then reverse the direction, going counter clockwise.

Allow your senses to become engulfed in the bodily sensations.

Create a healthy routine, one that will establish a new habit, such as daily face washing, exfoliating, using moisturizer, drink plenty of lemon water, and use sunscreen (free of chemicals).

Be sure to always read ingredient lists. Avoid artificial fragrances and use natural ingredients whenever possible.

Avoiding heavy perfumes and colognes will surprisingly, add years to your life.

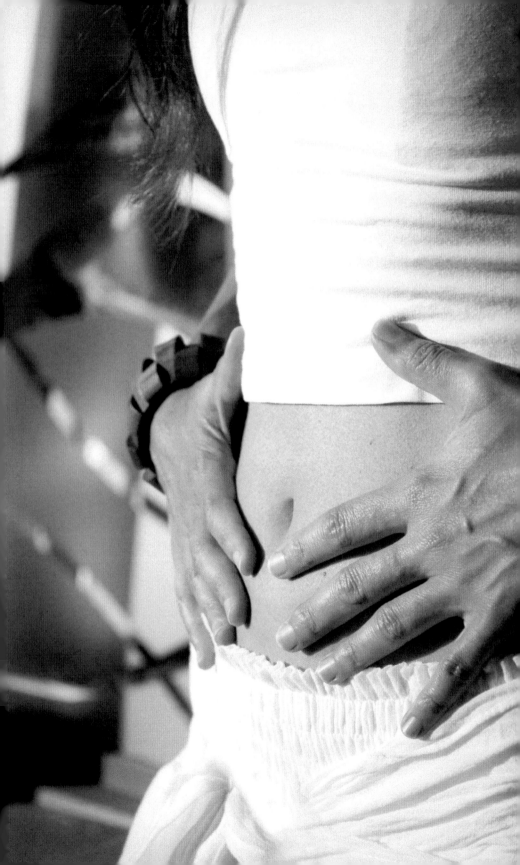

Looking at Yourself

When you look at yourself, what do you see?

What do you feel?

_____

_____

_____

_____

_____

_____

_____

_____

What do you know about yourself?

_____

_____

_____

_____

_____

_____

_____

What would you like to change?

What do you love about yourself?

The development of your body image begins in utero, yes, before you were even born.

The conscious and unconscious messages woven into your psyche, influence your perceptions and beliefs about your body.

The key development stage in our childhood is between birth and seven. This is the foundational stage of building the internal organs and the physical body.

It is during this time we are never more dependent in life than we are at birth and early years.

When you were born, your mother's liver sent a message and knowledge to your own, going back thousands of years in humankind's history, that it could take care of itself.

This message has been ingrained in our livers; however, we seldom offer them a helping hand as we go through life.

We are unaware of what the liver is doing for us, and it is completely on its own.

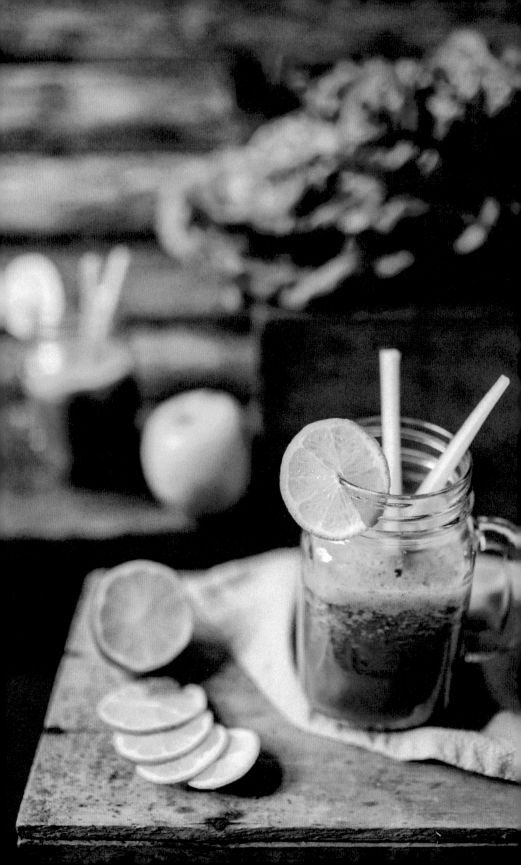

Until now... We can shift this course and do something about it. We can use our free will to make choices now that we are aware.

The liver does call out for love and when we simply think about the liver in a caring way, the spirit of the liver's immune system can feel it and even recharge from it.

Yes, I said the spirit of your liver. Our liver has a spirit. I cried when I found this out.

When we give our liver nourishment and nutrients like mineral-rich foods, we care for the liver and our liver's immune system strengthens.

Your liver's white blood cells carry intelligence.

While medical denial can keep us in the dark, we can play it smart by knowing that the liver's immune system is always kept in the light of knowing.

When we think about it, our lives are built on habits.

From which side of the bed you sleep on, morning tea, midnight snacks, or anything in between. Not all habits are negative, we can also create habits that are beneficial to our health.

The first step in creating any new habit is to make a decision to just do it!

Sometimes telling others helps keep you accountable, or having a family member, spouse or friend come along and do it together is the more desirable route. An accountability buddy.

Carving out time to commit to yourself is the greatest gift you can give yourself.

Create an affirmation such as "My body is a beautiful temple; I am full of energy and vitality."

Start visualising yourself starting to look and feel younger.

Believe and you shall receive.

How do you turn back the clock

and start to look

and feel

younger?

Remain open!

Nothing in life is by chance. You were led here for a reason. You seek the truth, your curiosity and desire to know has brought us together at this exact moment.

From the time you were born, you have learned skills to survive in this world.

You were influenced by two sets of people, family (parents) and teachers. Though you spent most of your time in school you were mostly influenced by your parents.

Do you remember the time your parents taught you to behave while out at a friend's house? Or the time you were reprimanded for not acting the way they wanted you to act?

Though they look like regular etiquette being told to us, these are examples of social conditioning.

This is to teach us to display acceptable behaviour in front of others.

Parenting is designed to bring up good values. Or perhaps you had less than favourable experiences.

Nonetheless, our parents inherited their values from their parents, traditions, religion, culture, or habits and passed them down from generation to generation.

Most never question or oppose them before adopting the behaviour.

There may have been judgements, false beliefs or ethical reasons.

This is a great hindrance to critical thinking or a free-thinking society.

Whatever outlook you bear towards life, our beliefs, relationships, our choices are all due to the influence of social conditioning since birth.

As adults, the fears we encounter are based on social acceptance. To a large extent, it leaves us powerless.

We are not meant to feel powerless, taking responsibility and acting on new found knowledge, influencing and working with people, this is our power.

One of the greatest gifts you can give is to share yourself and your love with your child. Set a time, and have date nights where you can have heart-to-heart meaningful conversations, sharing compassion, love and joy, being fully present, allowing your own inner child the opportunity to come out and play along the way.

When you show up in conscious ways for your child, you are setting a solid foundation for them, showering love and beauty, as the sunshine, food and medicine for a beautiful inner garden to flourish.

When you show up and share your love and time with others, whether it be your child, spouse, boss, or friend, you are showing up for yourself.

You will see that you are mirroring back all the love and beauty that you are, inside and out.

We all have a deep inner knowing, intuitiveness, a gut feeling.

A connection to the universe.

We are co-creators of our lives, but we cannot always control what happens.

Truth is, it's really not up to us to figure out.

Once you can detach from trying to control and plan life, and begin allowing and opening to life, you are no longer going to feel blocked, but instead, open to receive life's magical moments.

Now let's take a nice deep breath together and sigh it out. Ahhhhhh

Seed 2

How do I allow the body to work for me? How can I feel and look younger?

Beauty is not just skin deep.

What lies inside you is your key to whether you age or not.

A healthy liver is the ultimate anti-aging ally and ultimate de-stressor.

You look and feel younger by taking care of your liver!

The liver has everything to do with aging.

It's a big deal!

Snuggle in and get cosy, to discover the truth of what is going on inside our body.

The Liver's

Immune System

When we hear the term immune system, we usually think of the body's defence against fevers, colds, and sore throat.

Evidence of invaders isn't always as obvious as these symptoms though. Bacteria and viruses sometimes wage war and attack far beneath the surface, in our glands and organs.

More than we know, we rely on immune defences that happen deep beneath the surface to protect us from illnesses that have a much more lasting impact than the common cold.

The liver does not like bacteria and viruses residing inside of it, when it cannot stop them from entering, it does everything it can to keep them contained as deep within itself as possible.

The liver will send out killer cells after the viruses to keep them at bay and guard the deep internal fabric of the liver.

White blood cells are brought in randomly and periodically to control any viruses living deep within it.

When the virus tries to get out of the liver, special white blood cells are there to destroy it.

Why doesn't the liver send all of the white blood cells out to destroy all pathogens and viruses in the liver? The liver is already putting a huge number of resources trying to fight off new pathogens entering in through the hepatic portal vein and hepatic artery.

Trying to kill off the virus before entry so that they don't need to be buried in the liver in the first place.

Hepatic portal vein white blood cells monitor the portal vein itself. This is the main highway into the liver.

The hepatic portal white blood cells can survive being nearly suffocated from lack of oxygen and speed is not their game.

Blood coming from the hepatic portal vein is the path for the majority of the blood to the liver and comes unfiltered from the digestive tract; bacteria, viruses, pesticides from food eaten and everything else unproductive goes into your stomach, and, in turn, your intestinal tract can flow through this vein.

Specialized white blood cells stand watch over it all.

Hepatic artery white blood cells are stationed at the other circulatory entrance to the liver, the hepatic artery, because this blood is coming from the heart, it has higher levels of oxygen than the blood and travels at a higher velocity.

The white blood cells in the Hepatic artery are adapted to completely different oxygen levels and blood flow. Hepatic artery white blood cells must swim aggressively while worrying less about oxygen.

Pathogens that make it past the white blood cells, have to make it past the next layer of defence, lobule white blood cells.

Lobules border the capillaries and other blood vessels within the liver.

Your liver is your body's filter, it can be filled with any number of toxins.

Toxins such as heavy metal runoff, bacterial and viral waste, old pesticides like DDT muck up the liver, making it difficult for the lobule white blood cells to target active pathogens.

This is one of many reasons why keeping your liver clean and healthy is a critical part of protecting yourself from disease, not just liver disease, all disease.

Bile production is one of the top functions of your liver, there are special bile duct white blood cells assigned to watch over the bile duct system. These cells can withstand bile's harsh nature because they have protective covers, like firefighter's gear, undiscovered by medical science and research.

The bile duct white blood cells look for passers-by in the bile that may cause infection in the liver, duodenum, gallbladder, or intestinal tract, or travel farther up into the stomach.

Occasionally, a pathogen will slip by, at that point a signal will go out and a single bile duct white blood cell will launch a kamikaze attack, following the invader out of the liver into the duodenum, gallbladder and the rest of the small intestine, a path that will never let it return.

By the end of the journey, this path destroys and kills the bile duct white blood cell by burning away its protective cover.

Keep in mind there are not many of these blood cells, they are powerful, and the soul of our liver considers them heroic.

Finally, there are liver lymphocytes, that patrol the outer region of the liver. They are the "watchtower" positions in and around the lymphatic vessels there, they can also enter if necessary. They also have a license to kill, especially when they come upon Epstein-Barr Virus (EBV) cells trying to enter the liver through the lymph fluid and establish itself as a mono-nucleosis.

Liver lymphocytes also protect against other herpetic viruses such as human herpes virus 6 (HHV-6), (HHV-7), and the undiscovered HHV-10, HHV11, HHV 12, HHV13, HHV14, HHV15, and HHV16, the cofactor Streptococcus, various viral and bacterial mutations, and dangerous superbugs such as C. difficile and methicillin-resistant Staphylococcus aureus (MRSA).

When the liver is overburdened with toxins, from the environment and already present, viral load or unproductive foods that someone eats regularly, its filtration system gets backed up and these poisons often leach into the lymphatic system.

This makes the liver's lymphocytes job much harder. The watchtowers become saturated with poisons, and they are forced to leave. The lymphocytes travelling are also slowed down because the lymph fluid is filled with debris and sludge, and they cannot swim through it.

This can become treacherous because when pathogens such as EBV get into the lymphatic system they become very aggressive, in a war stage, trying to take up residency in organs such as the liver.

The pathogens will sometimes gang up on the lone lymphocytes and destroy them, winning the battle, though not the war, if you give your liver and lymphatic system the support they need.

We need our livers, and our livers need us. Knowing this is the missing piece of the puzzle.

When we treat the liver with intelligence, we assist it with the true miracle of healing.

When we combine our spiritual and physical, our liver's immune system can do the work it is meant to do.

If you push your liver too far, it slowly dies, before anything else does.

It slowly dies before the brain does, before we do.

It takes on the heat and the abuse.

It takes all of the hardship, and when you are under stress the liver ages fast, which in turn ages us.

When adrenaline is pumping and releasing hormones, fear, panic, fight or flight, the liver is soaking up these adrenaline batches to protect your life.

To keep you as young as possible.

Toxic environmental stuff we are dealing with, stress, and bad food choices create more work for the liver.

Eventually, the liver gets pushed over the edge, some people are maxed out by age twenty, long before we start to see weight gain, saggy skin, and age spots.

Why is it that someone can handle a lot of stress and not age, where as another mom will have a baby and it will hit her hard and age faster?

Why is this possible?

It is not the genes!

It's all about the liver. It's about having a healthier, better liver.

We all want to hold on to our youth, and stop aging, the answer is to not get distracted by false promises.

Tree — the apple — the Earth — the body and how the body uses that.

Giving thanks to mother Earth. We have lost that connection.

The forbidden fruit. What is fruit? What are the benefits of eating fruit?

Fruit is the divine word of wisdom. For thousands of years, we have used fruit to express powerful truths.

We use phrases such as "fruits of our labour", in business we talk about projects coming to "fruition".

All this fruit in our daily language shows how we connect on some level with fruit's significance.

For true mind-body-spirit-soul-heart wisdom, we need to incorporate real, unadulterated fruit into our diets.

When fruit literally becomes part of who we are, our lives become that much more fruitful.

Why avoid the food we were

most meant to eat?

Eating whole fruit can make us whole again.

Fruit has properties that help restore your adrenal glands, strengthen your entire endocrine system, repair your vascular system, restore, and cleanse your liver, help purge your lymphatic system, and revitalize your brain and stop it from atrophying.

There is no other food, no pill that enhances so many of your bodily functions as fruit.

You cannot function as a human being without glucose, the simple sugar into which your body breaks down foods.

Glucose fuels your liver, brain, your nervous system, and the cells throughout your body.

The highest quality source of sugar is fruit.

Fruits are made up of living water, minerals, vitamins, protein, fat, other nutrients, pulp, fibre, antioxidants, pectin and just a fraction of sugar.

Fruit is anti-cancerous!

Vegetables combat cancer too, but only about a quarter, as well as fruit does.

Incorporating an abundance of fruit into your diet will be a positive, proactive step toward countering and preventing cancer's effects.

Cancer cannot feed off of the sugar in fruit, which possesses critical components such as antibacterial, antiviral compounds and polyphenols and other antioxidants.

Fruits such as bananas, wild blueberries, apples, papaya, oranges, mangoes, and red pitaya (dragon fruit), are the most powerful natural destroyers of viruses on earth.

Fruit is vital for gut health, which is essential to a healthy immune system, because any pathogens, such as viruses and unproductive bacteria, that live inside the gut cannot thrive when you are eating enough fruit.

It's imperative that women eat enough fruit so they can avoid cancers, tumours, fatigue, viruses, and other illnesses.

It's important to the future of our children, who currently get the message not to eat fruit.

If you're in the business of wanting your liver, pancreas, and kidneys to break down, then go ahead and listen to advice to eat a high-fat, high-protein diet and shun fruit.

Fruit is a critical part of how you overcome illness, turn back the clock and reverse aging.

In truth, everything we do that helps our liver slows down and can reverse the aging process.

Magical Tools

LIVER RESCUE JUICE RECIPE

2 apples

2 cups coarsely chopped pineapple

1 inch ginger

1 bunch celery

1 cup loosely packed parsley

Run the apples, pineapple, ginger, celery, and parsley through a juicer.

Enjoy immediately for best results or store in an airtight container in the fridge.

LEAFY GREENS WITH AVOCADO DRESSING

For the salad

8 cups leafy greens (such as Romaine or cos lettuce, butter lettuce, spinach)

For the dressing

1 avocado

¼ cup water

5 sprigs fresh cilantro (coriander)

1 tablespoon lemon or lime juice

½ clove fresh garlic (or more to taste)

¼ teaspoon cayenne (optional)

Place leafy greens in a medium-sized bowl. Combine the avocado, water, cilantro, lemon or lime juice, garlic and cayenne in a blender and blend until very smooth. Add to the salad and toss until evenly coated.

Serve immediately.

HEALING BROTH RECIPES

Healing broth is a powerful, mineral-rich liquid that carries the essence of vitally nutritious vegetables, herbs, and spices in a way that is easy for the body to digest.

Healing benefits for both body and soul.

4 carrots, chopped or 1 sweet potato, cubed

2 stalks of celery, roughly chopped

2 onions, sliced

1 cup finely chopped parsley

1 cup shiitake mushrooms, fresh or dried (optional)

2 tomatoes, chopped (optional)

1 bulb garlic (about 8 cloves), minced

1-inch piece of fresh ginger, finely sliced, minced, or grated

8 cups water

1 hot chilli pepper or ½ teaspoon red pepper flakes (or more, to taste; optional)

Place all the ingredients in a pot and bring to a gentle boil. Turn the heat down to low and allow to simmer for about an hour. Strain and sip for a mineral-rich, healing, and restorative broth.

As an alternative, you can blend the broth with the vegetables for a pureed soup.

This recipe may be enjoyed as a chunky vegetable soup by leaving the vegetables whole within the broth.

TROPICAL FRUIT SALSA

½ ripe papaya, peeled, seeded, and cut into quarter-inch dice

¼ ripe pineapple, peeled, cored, and cut into quarter-inch dice

1 ripe mango, peeled, cored, and cut into quarter-inch dice

3 fresh figs, cut vertically into sixths (dried figs may be substituted if fresh are not available)

1 small red onion, peeled, cut into half-inch slices, charred over a flame, then chopped

1 red bell pepper, trimmed and cut into thin strips

Juice and minced zest of 1 lime

Juice and minced zest of 1 lemon

Juice and minced zest of 1 orange

I tablespoon finely chopped fresh mint

1 tablespoon finely chopped fresh cilantro

2 to 3 teaspoons peeled and minced ginger

Tablespoon raw honey

Pinch of salt

1. Combine all ingredients and season to taste. Set aside for 20 min while flavors meld.

Serve at room temperature or chilled.

Foods that are good for you

Lemon water - 16 oz room temperature, upon waking (½ a lemon)

Celery juice - 16 oz on an empty stomach for 20-30 min

Wild blueberries

Bananas

Apples

Oranges

Grapes

Spinach

Cilantro

Parsley

Tomatoes

Potatoes

Cucumbers

Asparagus

Kale

Ginger

Garlic

Papayas

Red pitaya

Lettuce

Foods to Avoid

Eggs

Dairy (including milk, cheese, butter, yoghurt, cream, and kefir[1])

Gluten

Soft drinks

---

1 fermented milk drink, cultured from kefir grains

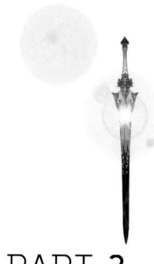

PART 2

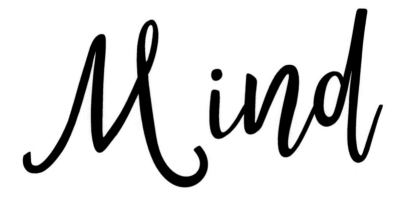

Mind

Seed 3

What resides in the Mind?

Not only is the social environment affecting your brain but also the environment inside you is shaping the human brain and the way you perceive the world and the life you are living.

Awareness is pivotal for mind health. Our ability to keep focus and move our attention voluntarily and resist distraction is key.

The ability to know what our mind is doing moment to moment and to make conscious choices about what our mind is doing. This awareness is expanding our view.

You can narrow the focus and pay attention primarily to a distraction, like someone interrupting you, and your frustration with the interruption. Or you can expand your focus to also include how you want to respond. If you are able to expand your awareness and pay attention to all three, you increase the likelihood that you will respond and not just react.

Having a caring connection is such an important part of maintaining a healthy lifestyle.

Maintaining interpersonal relationships with love, compassion, kindness, and appreciation is such a fundamental part.

A sense of safety, both psychological and physical is connected to how we relate to others. If you feel included in an upcoming party invite or dinner out with a friend, feeling valued, heard, and loved, you will be thriving.

However, if you sometimes feel ignored, unheard, banished, lonely or uncared for, you are in survival.

It is during this time that we speak gently with ourselves.

Give yourself a great big hug right now.

Our sense of connection is as important to our survival and well-being as food and water.

Understanding our inner dialogue and inner thoughts is so important. What stories do you tell yourself?

The way you think and the narratives you use are a constellation of your thoughts. This can be comforting or imprisoning you in your state of being.

Awareness is one way to notice if the stories you tell yourself are helpful or not.

Having a healthy mind includes having a sense of purpose and meaning. Having a strong sense of these makes you more resilient, you can recover from adversity more quickly.

It will allow you to put whatever difficulty you are facing into a larger context. The deeper the sense of meaning, the easier it will be to relate everyday activities to it.

Each interaction you have with others is an opportunity to practice awareness and a sense of connection.

Mindful meditation practices can strengthen brain circuitry and increase feel-good hormones such as serotonin. Paying attention in an open, accepting, non-judgmental way of yourself and allow whatever experience you are having in the moment.

As you pay attention to what your mind is doing, allow feelings of compassion and kindness for yourself and others, noticing but not getting lost in the stories and reconnecting with purpose.

Staying present and being in the moment allows your mind to be right there with you. Look around you and see what you see, smell any scents, hear the sounds, and take it all in.

Take a deep breath to help ground yourself and relax.

If you start to pay attention and notice what you have to be grateful for, you will start seeing more and more of it around you.

Like attracts like, be sure to focus on the good in your life.

When you are having thoughts the best thing you could do is put it down on paper. Journaling helps the brain release and relax. It helps quiet the mind.

If you know you may have to engage with someone who triggers an unfavourable response then plan accordingly and try to avoid going directly into the fire. If you know the person is unavoidable, then I suggest you pay attention to your breath and when you are tempted to respond, pause, then take a deep breath instead.

When you are having thoughts that keep running through your mind you can release their power. Talk to a friend, hearing the words out loud can diffuse the angst and help you move forward.

One of my all-time favorite things to do is listen to music. Listening to upbeat tunes will surely get you out of your head.

Allow yourself to go to a magical land with cool running water, engage your senses as if you are actually there.

Take deep cleansing breaths and allow the scene to quiet your mind, coming back refreshed with clear thinking.

We can loosen our attachments, beginning with our mind and its opinions and beliefs, which are based on good or bad.

There is no good or bad.

There is choice, and with each behaviour we have consequences.

We tend to get so serious about life, me included. It becomes a layer of constriction for many. Some of us get caught up in science, politics, or religion. We get bogged down in our own seriousness.

We are here to learn, to loosen our grip within the illusion, and to realise that death is a falsehood. We can change our view and begin to act and think selflessly.

Delight comes with only a beginner's mind. Start to look at life through the eyes of a child.

Begin to look at life with awe and wonder again.

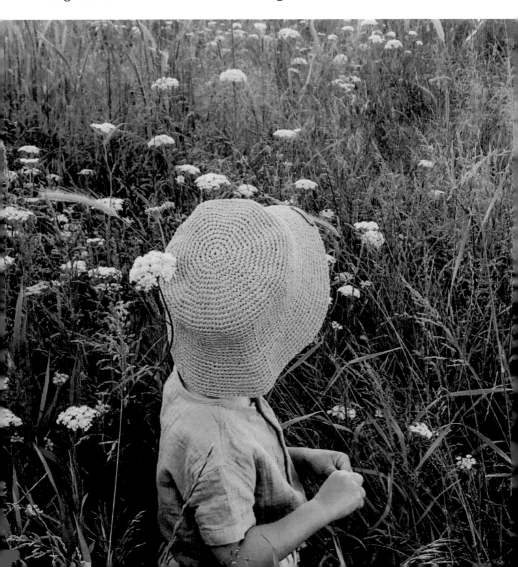

Seed 4

How to Quiet the Mind

Do you get lost in your thoughts?

Does your mind wander often when you are trying to focus?

Do you wish you could quiet your thoughts so you can think more clearly?

One of your greatest tools is your breath.

When you feel overwhelmed, stressed, or anxious your body temperature rises and your heart rate increases.

Taking long, slow, deep breaths can help you physically relax.

Start by breathing in for three seconds, hold for four seconds and breathe out for five seconds. When your out-breath is longer than your in-breath, you reduce the activation of your stress state and encourage your body to move into a thrive state.

If you are feeling any physical tension, you can draw attention to the body part that is sore or tight and tighten that area and then release it a few times until you feel relaxed.

Self-soothing touch and discovery is very therapeutic,

A good way to do the practice is to start from your head and end at your toes. Try this lying down before you go to sleep. Ideally, by the time you get to your feet, you are relaxed or asleep.

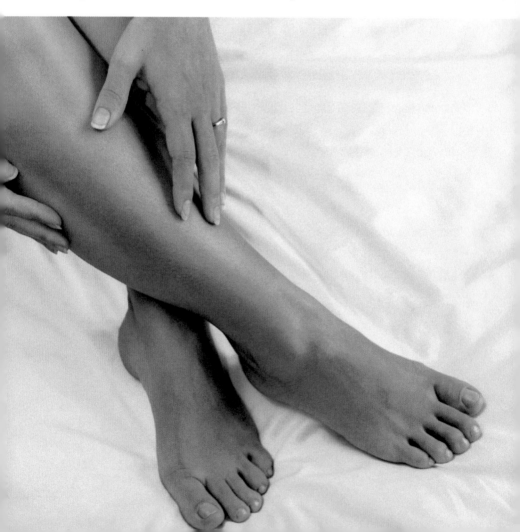

Seed 5

Ways to cleanse the Mind

When cleansing your mind, it is also good to let go of thoughts and emotions that you have unconsciously blocked from coming to the surface. One option is to write a letter to someone who has hurt you or let you down. Use the letter to explain how their actions made you feel. You don't have to send it!

The point is to gain a better understanding of emotions you may have suppressed unknowingly. Let them escape from your body, so they no longer harm you or age you.

Another way to cleanse is to keep a journal. Allow yourself a set time when you sit down and dedicate time to yourself. Seek to understand how you feel instead of pushing these feelings away. Use this as a way to move forward, leaving the undesirable thoughts and feelings behind.

Have you ever thought to put your phone down?

How about setting a time throughout the day when you put the phone down? Give your body a break.

When the phone does ring and you have to answer it, I suggest you put the call on speaker so that the sound waves are not going from the tower straight to the side of your head.

When you look around at your surroundings, take note.

Get rid of your clutter!

Think of the clutter around you as your brain, and as you tidy your surroundings up, you are also cleaning and opening up space in your brain, which in turn will reflect in your life.

The number of things in your surroundings that are not being used or enjoyed can go bye-bye. Donate it then to your local charity.

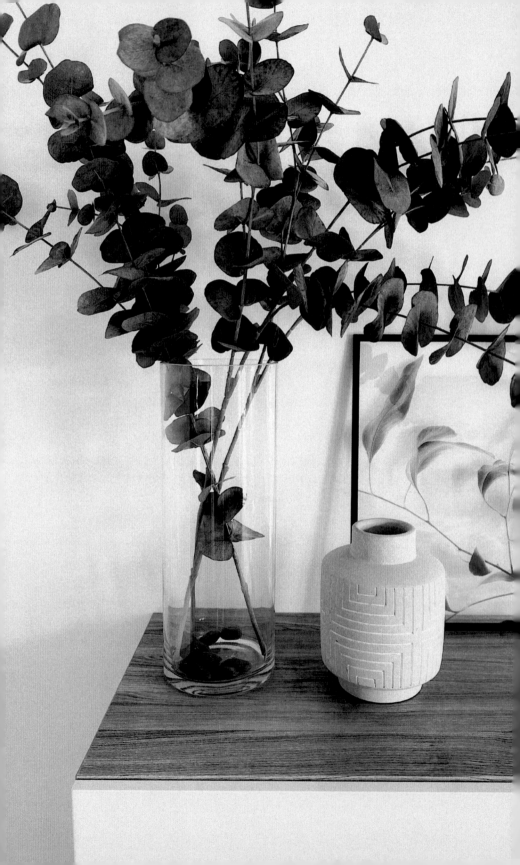

The top three nutritional components that your brain relies upon are trace mineral salts, glucose, and vitamin B12.

With our trace mineral salt and glucose reserves low, our brain fire burns high because adrenaline takes over and becomes the fuel for our electrical grid.

If we don't have enough glucose to cool down the brain when we're up against emotional struggle, our brain tissue can get scorched, leading to calluses and scar tissue.

We literally experience burnout.

The brain can heal and recover and return. It takes time and appreciation for how our brain really works.

Electrical conductors are another important part of brain function. Electrolytes serve as these conductors in your brain, and trace mineral salts are the building blocks of those electrolytes.

Trace mineral salts are part of the foundation of your brain.

Trace minerals in the brain are more critical than essential fatty acids. Electricity cannot run through brain tissue without trace mineral salts. These trace mineral salts are not to be confused with adding salt to food.

Rock salt and sea salt do not remedy the trace mineral deficiency problem. These salts' composition is changed because they have been isolated and separated from their natural environment. These salts are too concentrated.

We get the best, most bioavailable trace mineral salts from healing sources such as lemons and celery juice.

Neurotransmitter hormones need trace minerals in order to be complete. They work side by side.

Deficiencies of trace minerals inside the brain lead to temporary relapses of any type of symptom and condition as electrical activity drives through patchy spots of brain tissue in areas where trace minerals are deficient. Those patchy spots become part of the electrical highway of the brain where electricity dims down.

This creates inconsistency, causing someone to struggle, whether in receiving information or expressing themselves, delivering information vocally or writing it. Toxic heavy metals and viral neurotoxins in the brain worsen the effects of this deficiency.

The fewer trace minerals in the brain, the hotter brain tissue becomes, because trace minerals control heat in the brain, while glucose cools down the brain.

If someone is very deficient, void of many trace mineral salts and therefore electrolytes, it can almost feel like it hurts when they think too hard.

That's because brain cells near the electrical current pathway heat up excessively from the transmission of information, because trace minerals are not present, causing a person to shut down.

Key trace minerals in the brain help support us in believing in ourselves.

We tend to think that managing our thoughts is the answer to burnout. Controlling our brain waves, our neurological pathways, with positive thoughts and meditation is believed to be the key to solving burnout. And yes, that can be helpful.

Mental practices only get us so far on their own. Lasting relief comes from addressing supply and demand deficiencies in the brain and factors that drain our brains faster than we can replenish them.

Toxic heavy metals are a leading cause of today's epidemic of brain deterioration, dysfunction, and disease.

Toxic heavy metals are also passed along through our bloodline via metal contaminated egg and sperm, so generation after generation comes into this world with inherited heavy metals such as Mercury.

Toxic heavy metals are behind most life-altering brain-related conditions of our time.

Symptoms such as depression, OCD, and Alzheimer's. Toxic heavy metals are also behind many of the daily challenges and frustrations, from anger issues to anxiousness to focus and concentration issues and brain fog.

The brain can accumulate heavy metals through the brain's electromagnetic field, which is meant to draw in beneficial trace minerals.

Just in case you might be feeling sceptical about how toxic heavy metals even find their way into our bodies in the first place, picture a ball of aluminium foil and think how could that find its way inside me?

Well, by touch, and when we pick up a can or wear copper-based jewelry, oils from our hands and skin, extract and absorb minute levels of the metals, drawing them into our derma and then deeper into our system.

Oil is extremely acidic, and that acidic nature reacts to metal. An acidic chemical interaction occurs, forcing the metal to release metal by-product molecules.

We ingest toxic heavy metals too.

Herbicides, pesticides, and fungicides.

Pharmaceuticals have some levels of toxic heavy metals in them as well.

Plug-in air fresheners and scented candles.

Toxic heavy metals support viruses in their mission to elevate inflammation throughout the body and cause auto-immune conditions. Taking metals away helps lower the viral load.

Extracting heavy metals also addresses mental and emotional struggles and well-being by allowing the electricity and energetic frequencies of the brain to flow freely.

When you break down and dismantle the alloys that have interfered with your brain, you minimize viral invasion, allow for emotional injuries to heal faster, reduce inflammation of the brain and cranial nerves, address burnout and deficiencies, and help relieve an addicted, acid brain.

A key to safeguarding yourself and your loved ones is acknowledgement.

Magical Tools

16 oz room temp lemon water upon waking (½ a lemon)

16 oz organic celery juice on an empty stomach 20-30 min

HEAVY METAL DETOX SMOOTHIE

2 Bananas

2 cups frozen or fresh wild blueberries, or 2 oz pure wild blueberry juice,

or 2 tablespoons pure wild blueberry powder

1 cup tightly packed fresh cilantro (coriander)

1 teaspoon barley grass juice powder

1 teaspoon spirulina

1 tablespoon atlantic dulse or 2 dropperfuls atlantic dulse liquid

1 orange, juiced

1/2 to 1 cup water, coconut water, or additional fresh squeezed orange juice (optional)

Combine the bananas, wild blueberries, cilantro, barley grass juice powder, spirulina, atlantic dulse with the juice of 1 orange in a high-speed blender and blend until smooth.

Add up to 1 cup of water, coconut water, or orange juice if a thinner consistency is desired.

Serve and enjoy!

If you are using coconut water, make sure that it does not contain natural flavors and is not pink or red in colour.

Children will greatly benefit; portion size will vary.

Think about how much they usually drink with orange juice. For example 6-8 ounces. That is an appropriate amount to give a child. You cannot overdose on too much yummy goodness.

Recommended supplement site, www.vimergy.com for Barley Grass Juice Powder, Spirulina, and Atlantic Dulse. I personally order all my supplements from this A+++ family-owned company.

Meditation

As we are together, praying for peace, let us be truly with each other.

Let us pay attention to our breathing.

Let us be relaxed in our bodies and our minds.

Let us be at peace with our bodies and our minds.

Let us return to ourselves and become wholly ourselves.

Let us maintain a half-smile on our faces.

Let us be aware of the source of being common to us all and to all living things.

Evoking the presence of the Great Compassion, let us fill our hearts with our own compassion towards ourselves and towards all living beings.

Let us pray that all living beings realize that they are all brothers and sisters, all nourished from the same source of life.

Let us pray that we ourselves cease to be the cause of suffering to each other.

Let us plead with ourselves to live in a way which will not deprive other beings of air, water, food, shelter, or the chance to live.

With humility, with awareness of the existence of life, and of the sufferings that is going on around us, let us pray for the establishment of peace in our hearts and on earth. Amen

THICH NHAT HANH

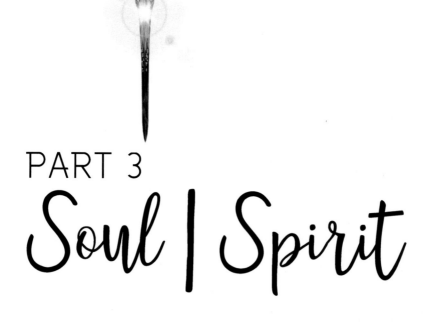

PART 3
Soul | Spirit

Seed 6

What is God?

I know how I feel about God, I know my truth about what GOD is for me.

We are all so uniquely different, and for that reason, life is so enjoyable, in so many glorious ways.

What is God for you?

God is believed by some, to be the eternal, all knowing, supreme being who created and preserves all things.

God is all present.

Yes, is God's favorite and most repeated word. Mostly it is spoken in the Hebrew form, amen.

The Hebrews said amen where we would say yes.

I much prefer the word yes, myself.

If someone asks me, would I like this or that? My response is I would like this and that.

I've started implementing this practice into my life, try it, it feels amazing.

Spirit of the Most High, God's expression of compassion, whom Anthony William, Medical Medium calls Spirit of Compassion, came into his life when he was four years old. He speaks to him as if a friend were standing beside him.

For those of you who are fearful or put off by the word, medium, keep in mind that the voice is outside his ear, it's an independent source separate from his thoughts. He is different, Spirit is distinct and separate from him. Anthony said, "It is like having someone follow him around everywhere."

Spirit of Compassion sees the human condition on this planet and then provides a deep understanding of how it came to be, why, and what to do here on earth.

Anthony, at age 8, asks, Spirit of the Most High, "What are you? Who are you? Where did you come from? And why are you here?"

Spirit replied, "First I will tell you what I am not. "I am not a person. And I am not an Angel. I was never a human being. I am not a 'spirit guide,' either.

"I am a word."

Spirit replied, "Compassion."

"Spirit are you God?"

"No," the voice replied. "At the fingertip of God sits a word, and that word is compassion. I am that word. A living word. The closest word to God.

Anthony asked, how can you be just a word? "A word is an energy source. Certain words hold great power. God pours light into words such as I and instils us with the breath of life.

I am more than a word.

Anthony asked, "Is there anyone like you?" He asked.

"Yes: Hope, Faith, Joy, Peace, And more. They are all living words, but I sit above all of them, because I am the closest to God."

He continued to ask Spirit, "Do these words speak to people, too?

"Not as I do to you Anthony. These words are not heard by the ear. They live in each person's heart and soul. As do I.   Words such as joy and peace do not stand alone in the heart. They require compassion to be complete".

"Why can't peace be enough by itself?" Anthony asks.

"Compassion is the understanding of suffering," Spirit replies.

"There is no joy, peace, or hope until those who suffer are understood. Compassion is the soul of these words: without it, they are empty. Compassion fills them with truth, honour, and purpose.

"I am Compassion. And no other sits above me but God."

Anthony trying to make sense of this, asked, "Then what is God"?

"God is a word. God is Love, which is above all other words. God is also more than a word. Because God loves all. God is the most powerful source of existence.

"People can love. But people do not love all others unconditionally, God does."

"The Angels and other beings look to me for guidance. I provide all who care to listen with the lessons and wisdom of God, "Spirit says.

God loves us loyally, unconditionally, and perfectly.

God's love is unconditional, gracious, merciful, and patient.

I work for the light; I work for God.

Bridging the Soul and the Spirit

You enter the world as an energy, totally open and aware.

The school of life is the place where you are given an opportunity to learn.

The process of learning makes the journey more interesting and gives you a chance to evolve.

The crisis years and times of drastic transformations in life are the lessons offered by the universe.

How well you manage to implement the solutions to challenges in life determines if you pass the exams.

You are offered chances to advance in life, being open to opportunities as they are presented.

A key to having a successful spiritual cycle is opening up your inner connection and following what you feel is best.

As you sense what you truly desire and do what you can, you will be learning and experiencing what you need throughout your life journey.

Nature has taught us everything we know. To reach harmony in life, we all need to learn how to observe nature and learn the laws that govern our universe.

If you are following the mission of your higher self, there is no need to be afraid of the times in life when lessons are being learned. It is a chance for our soul to grow and evolve.

Listen to your own intuition and trust your inner compass.

A fun exercise to do is make a list of all the things that give you pleasure and motivate you in life.

How do they make you feel happy?

_____

_____

_____

_____

_____

_____

_____

_____

What brings you joy and love?

_____

_____

_____

_____

_____

_____

_____

Answering these questions will give you a window inside yourself.

Find that magical place, where you feel alive and full of excitement.

What lights your soul on fire?

Our soul purpose is to remember the truth of who we are, and then share that with the world.   It can be as simple as a smile.

According to most, your soul does exist. Everyone has a soul. It is the voice of your entire existence.

Your soul holds knowledge of all the events that have occurred in your life. Your soul is a record that contains the meaning of your physical existence.

Your soul harnesses every single journey you have experienced or chosen in a physical living form.

Your soul lives forever and sustains itself, long after the physical part of you has perished.

It doesn't matter if you like your soul, love your soul, or hate your soul. It does not matter if you believe in the soul's existence or believe you have a soul. It does not matter because your soul is more powerful than you, more powerful than your consciousness in your present state of being.

Your soul is more powerful than any form of manipulation or brainwashing you have been conditioned with here on earth because your soul has been far away from the earth, and is not governed in this earthbound bubble of our human-created environment.

Your soul is much more than you.

It is your light.

A light from above that did not start here on earth.

Your soul is much older than your physical body and has memories and information from the past to which you do not have conscious access.

Your soul has the power to lead you on your way even when it's underfed and broken by the people around you or the world we live in.

Your soul's leftover fragments still hold the power and the glory that brighten the way on the darkest path.

When we voice ourselves here on earth, sometimes we find moments when we transcend the confusion here, and what we're speaking is more than just our own truth; it is a common truth that unites us with others, one that may even go beyond words. This can be our true, powerful voice.

Many times, truth can be flawed here on earth.

Your soul holds authentic truth, pure and untainted, regardless of any survival mechanisms we have to use here on earth.

Your true soul always knows better and is wiser than the truth games played here on earth.

This truer voice is elevated above the voice we know to come from a deep place within, because as strong and deep as our earthly voice is, it is often mixed with sorrow and hurt.

The truest voice we possess cannot be swayed by trickery. It resides inside all of us. It is your soul.

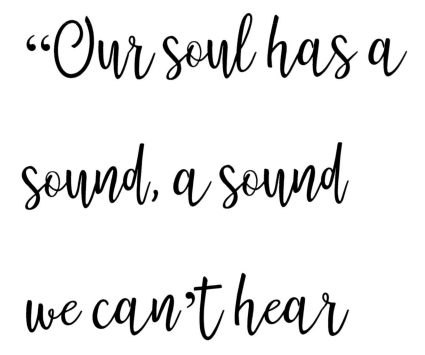

"Our soul has a sound, a sound we can't hear

with our physical ears, a sound that rings true through time and space."

ANTHONY WILLIAM, MEDICAL MEDIUM

When our soul leaves our physical body and transcends upward, there is a noise made, a sound.

The soul is energy, and the soul's energy is powerful. It's described as a fireball of light.

As the soul travels, the sound is the noise of the soul piercing time itself, for time no longer exists for the soul once the soul has left the body.

There is no clock where the soul goes.

Spirit continues on saying that the home our soul goes back to cannot be governed by time because time is different for every planet, every galaxy, and every solar system.

If one planet or solar system ceases to exist, then time stops for that planet or solar system, yet our soul cannot cease to exist.

Our soul needs to live on, and it does, without constraints of time.

Our soul is an energy force that isn't constrained by what happens here on earth, it is a universal, God-conceived law that our soul has it right and safely right, even if our consciousness connected to our brain has it wrong.

Wrong cannot enter and destroy a soul.

What really matters in the end is the truth of the soul because it is our forever existence.

Seed 7

How the Soul and Spirit connects to the Heart

Everyone is unique and different. Each person's soul is different too.

If I ask you,

What pain do you want in your life?

What are you willing to struggle for?

What is the pain that you want to sustain?

This question can change your life. It's what makes me, me, and you, you. It's what defines and separates us, and ultimately brings us together.

Who you are is defined by the values you are willing to struggle for. People who enjoy the struggles of the gym are the ones who get in good shape.

People who enjoy the stresses and uncertainty of the starving artist life are ultimately the ones who live it and make it.

Our willpower is our spirit.

The soul, heart, and spirit are three entirely different components of one's being that always get grouped together.

The soul is the consciousness of a person, or what some call "the ghost in the machine."

According to Spirit, your soul resides in your brain, where your soul stores your memories and experiences. When you pass from this mortal realm, your soul carries those memories as it moves onward. Even if a person has a brain injury or disease that keeps them from remembering certain things, the soul will bring all the memories with it when that person passes. Your soul also stores your faith and your hope, both of which help keep you on the right path.

As I read all of this for the first time, personally, my soul was gleaming with excitement. I was jumping up and down with such delight. As I am now, inside, knowing that you too are hearing this information.

Intermission, dance party time!!!!

Sing Along...

I've got the joy, joy, joy, joy, down in my heart, (where?) Down in my heart, (where?) Down in my heart. I've got the joy, joy, joy, joy Down in my heart (where?) Down in my heart to stay.

Ideally, you should have a fully intact soul. Traumatic events such as betrayal by a loved one or betrayal of self, death of a loved one, can cause the soul to become fractured according to Spirit.

A person with soul damage is vulnerable. Not being ready for another relationship, still hurting from a breakup, needs time before risking putting themselves out there again.

Another example is hungrily pursuing spiritual learning in any form, it may be because that person's soul has been damaged, and she or he is instinctively searching for ways to make it healthy and complete again.

Spirit says, "That's a critical job for each of us, when your time here ends, your soul should be sufficiently intact to survive its journey beyond the stars, where God will receive it".

The physical heart is the other component of one's being. This is where love, compassion and joy reside.

Having a healthy soul does not necessarily make you a whole person.

You can have an unblemished soul and a broken, injured heart.

The heart serves as the compass for your actions, helping to guide you to do the right thing when your soul becomes lost.

The heart is also the safety net that can compensate for soul damage.

Guess what? Your heart keeps a record of your good intentions, too.

This means that you can have a warm, loving heart and a battered soul. It is common for someone's heart to grow larger as a result of the ups and downs his or her soul has gone through.

Deep understanding and a greater love and compassion come from great losses.

A person's spirit is their will and physical strength.

Your soul is not your spirit. They are two separate parts of you.

Your willpower helps you fight, even if your soul's been battered and your heart is faint, your willpower keeps you going, while you look for opportunities to heal.

Spirit shared, that in order to be a compassionate healer, you have to adapt to each unique condition and personality to alleviate that person's pain and suffering.

This compassion is the most important element in healing.

Seed 8

What are Angels?

Angels are everywhere, open up to them and allow them to communicate with you.

Music is a universal language and Angels use song to convey messages in various ways, often communicated through reoccurring songs.

Make it a daily practice to listen to music, feel free to sing your heart out, let it all go.

Have fun and smile!

Have you ever noticed a particular smell, shape or sound and have been unable to identify the source? This may show up in the form of a lovely sweet scent.

We often question our 6th sense, so they send messages perceptible through smells, sights and sounds.

Angel shapes in the clouds, flickering lamps, and finding feathers along your walk are signs Angels are near.

Over the years I have collected many beautiful feathers that I display throughout my house, which bring so much inner happiness, I smile often when I pass by.

This is often a sign that Angels are bringing encouragement and validation from heaven.

This is often a confirmation of your intuition.

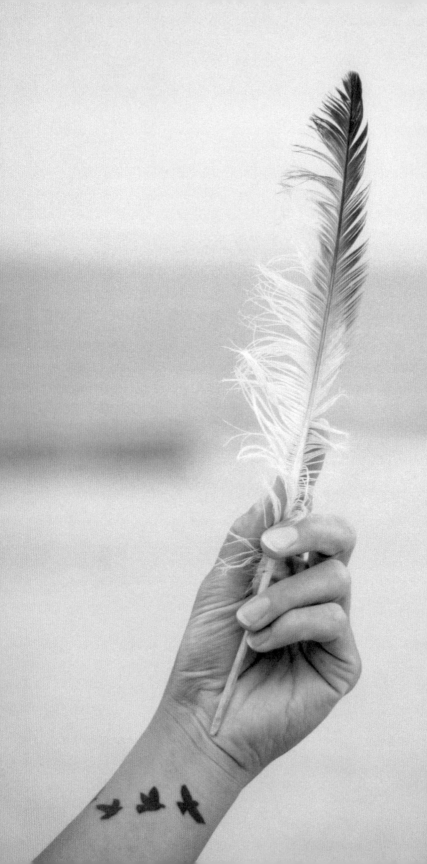

The scent of roses or flowers are often a sign Angels are around to help calm and lift your spirits.

If you notice a rainbow, this is a sign that Angels are bringing encouragement and validation from heaven.

Has a bright star in the sky ever caught your eye or a bright orb nearby? These are signs Angels are near. Stop and breathe for a moment and allow their angelic presence to bring you healing and uplift you, feeling lighter and younger.

Do you feel a special connection with your house pets or volunteer at a shelter?

It is a magical and unique way to connect with an animal's soul.

Animals sense our emotions and respond with love, acceptance and comfort.

We receive a profound sense of being seen, heard and felt.

Animals don't ask for much, they seek your presence and offer excitement with doggie kisses and tail wags.

My dearest Angel friend, Lisa Jacenich has always shared with me and our tribal friends the saying, 'puppy pile.'

We all come together and layer up on one another.

Snuggling, giggling, and making beautiful memories together.

The next time you find yourself around friends, engage in a puppy pile.

Give a great big hug and relax in the comfort of knowing you are loved.

Earth Angels are empathic and sympathetic with others since they feel other people's energy and emotions as if they were there's.

Have you heard your whole life, "You're so sensitive?"

Turns out this is indeed one of your greatest gifts.

Your ability to be compassionate and understanding could mean people open up to you easily and you create intimacy with new people quickly, having friends with many different world views from different backgrounds.

Friendships promote longevity and laughter increases feel good hormones, adding years to your life.

Nature Earth Angels work with the energy of nature and are guardians of nature and our food supply.

Working to create a more green world and sustainable world will fill you with energy and purpose, you will feel calmer, grounded and expansive.

Look into creating a community garden and come together to harvest fresh fruits and vegetables.

Get grounded in Mother Earth, get your hands and feet in the dirt, connect with the birds, bees, and insects. Align your body rhythms to that of nature.

Allow yourself time to play and be full of ideas, creative projects and creative outlets such as an outdoor retreat, your body will thank you by feeling relaxed and refreshed after just a few short hours.

When you meet up with friends and family shortly after, they will ask, what have you done differently with yourself? You look younger and refreshed.

Did you know?

Angels attempt to get your attention and guide you through numbers. You may be sitting behind a car with 333 on its license plate or look at the clock every day at 11:11 exactly. If you are wondering what the point of seeing these numbers over and over again is all about, think of signs they leave as an endless possibility of growth and transformation.

Each number will have its own significance for you, and over time you will start to see the patterns and revelations will occur more often.

Now that you understand how to spot the signs that Angels are around you, what should you do with this new awareness?

Upon waking in the morning, spend a moment and feel gratitude, boost your vibration and align your frequency to feelings of bliss and elevate yourself to a state of positivity that constantly attracts more of the same.

These feelings will communicate on a deep level to your cells to promote wellness and youthfulness.

Remain open and share your light with others.

For every Angel fluttering through the skies, there is a divine counterpart here on earth.

Each of us has

a golden

celestial-self

just waiting to

be awakened.

Sue K.

Be an Angel, God loves a helping hand.

Every great dream begins with a dreamer. Always remember, you

have within you

the strength, the

patience, and

the passion to

reach for the

stars to change the world.

Harriet Tubman

You were born with the God given right to reach out to Angels whenever you may need them.

Angels want to help ease our mind, heal our body, our spirit and soul.

They want to direct us in our most purposeful direction.

Angels have existed since humankind began, to help us adapt to challenges and survive.

Angels are powerful partners, especially during times of change.

During these times or any time for that matter, you can call upon the Angels and they would be more than happy to assist.

The word "Angels" is derived from the Greek term angelos, which means "messenger" or "envoy".

Angels are the messengers of the divine.

They were created by the divine and are not matter, they are more light.

You can ask them for assistance any time, day, or night.

Talk to the Angels, the same way you would call a friend or loved one, knowing that you are never alone.

The Angels are here to help us with our decision-making, and to make the most of our free will.

The Angels are here to present opportunities and intercept trouble.

Angels do not exist to fulfil our every wish and desire; they are here to help us do God's work.

The secret is that you have to know the right Angels to ask, you have to have faith, you have to be open, and you have to work with them.

The three basic facts that you have to understand about Angels is that they work for God, their powers are vast, but infinite, and they have free will.

The 21 essential Angels, that I am sharing with you now, are critical for your times of need.

The number 21 stands for rebirth, new beginnings, and fresh starts.

Each Angel is potent and powerful. You can always call one or as a team.

It is important to know, you have to ask for their help aloud, if you are deaf, have a speech impairment, or are too weak to speak, then use sign language or your thoughts to ask for the Angel of Deliverance. She will express your soul's wishes to the other Angels.

This is the secret truth that will change your relationship with Angels.

Don't be afraid to ask the angelic forces for help with your problems. You do not have to frame your requests in only positive terms, or only use affirmations. You are not perpetuating the negative in your life by saying, I am desperate for help, or my body is weak, you are just stating the facts.

You are showing great honesty and strength by accepting the truth in your life and wanting to move forward.

You get to heal and have good things happen to you. Tapping into the Angel's power, your life will change.

Angel of Mercy

In your darkest hour, more powerful than the archangels. She is one of the strongest Angels in God's angelic realm. God has summoned her many times to battle darkness.

Angel of Faith

Call upon in any way that suits you. Call on daily to allow the rhythm to transition the habit into full-blown conviction.

Angel of Trust

When you are struggling to recover from a betrayal.

Angel of Healing

To provide temporary relief and heal a loved one. For longer relief, you must call on other Angels to help build you up to a point where you can heal yourself.

Angel of Restitution

Helps you recover from emotional trauma and resolve deep-seated issues.

Angel of Deliverance

Provides relief to someone going through an earthly judgement.

Angel of Sun

Call for her while in the sun to open up your body's cells so they can fully take in the healing power of the rays.

Angel of Light

Name her in order to be bathed in restorative angelic light given to her by God. The Angel of Light is more powerful than any light on earth, and more powerful even than the light of the sun.

Angel of Water

You can ask her to change the frequency of the water you bathe in to make it more cleansing, grounding and nourishing. If you are soaking a wound, you can call upon her to quicken its healing.

Angel of Air

After an encounter such as an argument, ask the Angel of Air to cleanse the negative vibration that person passed onto you. This is a powerful technique to change your frame of mind.

Angel of Purity

When you want to rid yourself of an addiction, this Angel can help you break free from the poisonous chains of habit.

Angel of Fertility

For aid in conception and carrying a baby to term.

Angel of Birth

For mother and child's health during birth.

Angel of Peace

To help heal your mental distress and bring new seeds of positivity and hope.

Angel of Beauty

If you feel closed off to the beauty of nature that surrounds you, trees, sun, and rivers, summon the Angel of Beauty. This Angel is your ally when a romantic partner is obsessed with talking about people's physical appearance when a co-worker's good looks have turned him vain, or a sibling's physical beauty earns her all the attention. Ask the Angel of Beauty to shift people's mindsets to recognize true beauty - the beauty of a shining soul.

Angel of Purpose

Call upon her if you are struggling with your purpose here on earth. If you have lost confidence in something or everything, the Angel of Purpose will be by your side.

Angel of Knowledge

When a loved one needs advice and you are at a loss, or you want to give more than a pat on the back, you'd be surprised at the healing, soothing words that come out of your mouth when you call upon this Angel. If you need advice or information and don't know where to find it, call on the Angel of Knowledge.

Angel of Wisdom

For guidance when you are about to make a big decision.

Angel of Awareness

To help you stay fully present in the moment. Also, if you want the people around you to be less judgemental and better communicators, you can call upon this Angel to help open their minds.

Angel of Relationships

If you are having a problem with someone you are dating or your spouse, or if you are single and looking for a good match.

Angel of Dreams

You can ask her to enter your dreams and help sort out and resolve emotional turmoil. Even if your waking life is troubled, call upon her to help you re-experience that soul freedom in your dreams.

There are also 144,000 Unknown Angels that do not have names. This is the holy number that God reveres.

Since they are unnamed, they have no notoriety and very little temptation to develop an ego. The unknown Angels are some of the most powerful of all, and the least in demand.

If you have faith in them, they can perform miracles. They do their work on you when you are asleep, restoring both your soul and body.

Miracles happen all around us; we just have to be open to receiving.

Magical Tools

SANSKRIT

Guess what? I speak Sanskrit!

What is Sanskrit?

The earliest form of Sanskrit is that used in the Rig Veda. It is considered the language of the gods; it literally means perfected.

It is recognized as both a classical language and an official language, with its oldest texts dating back to around 1500-500 B.C.

Sanskrit is probably the second oldest language in the world still being used today.

We often hear the word "vedanta" in yoga classes, meditation groups and spiritual gatherings.

What is Vedanta and where does it come from?

"Veda" means complete knowledge and "anta" means end. Vedanta means the culmination of Vedic wisdom or the final step on our spiritual journey.

The Vedas are said to be divine knowledge, that is heard from a divine source.

The ancient wisdom tradition of Vedanta examined the various sounds produced in nature and the vibrations of the world around us.

According to Vedanta, these sounds are an expression of infinite or cosmic mind and provide the basis for every human language.

If you sound out all the letters of the alphabet, the consonants, and the vowels, you will hear that these are the same sounds that all babies make spontaneously.

These sounds also contain the same vibrations that animals make, and if you listen carefully, you will notice that these sounds are everywhere in nature.

These are the sounds of thunder, wind, fire crackling, and ocean waves crashing on the shore.

Nature is vibration. Vibration is how infinite potential expresses itself.

All things are made up of vibration and each vibration interacts with vibration.

We interpret that as matter and sensation.

Mantra is a sacred word that describes this quality to the universe, a word, sound, or phrase, often in Sanskrit.

Your body is constantly vibrating, but the sounds of vibration are so subtle that you usually don't hear them.

We can all hear the same vibrations any time. If you sit quietly, when there is no noise around, you will hear a hum in the air.

If you start paying attention to that background hum, with practice you will actually end up hearing all the mantras that have been recorded in the Vedic literature.

The Vedas say that if you say a mantra out loud, its special pattern of vibrations creates its own effects, and can create events in our current physical realm.

Reciting the mantra mentally creates a mental vibration, which then becomes more abstract.

Ultimately it takes you into the field of pure consciousness or spirit from where the vibration arose.

A mantra is a very good way to transcend and go back to the source of thought, which is pure consciousness.

Each mantra produces its own, unique, specific vibration.

The mantra I use, and recommend for achieving miracles, is the mantra "so-hum".

This is the mantra of the breath. As you breathe, you make the sound so-hum, as air moves in and out of your lungs.

As you inhale, the sound of that vibration is "so". And as you exhale, the sound becomes "hum".

If you want, you can experiment with this. Inhale deeply, close your eyes and your mouth, and exhale forcefully through your nose. If you concentrate, you will hear the "hum" sound clearly.

One technique of meditation is focusing on the breath and where the breath comes from.

With your eyes closed, inhale and think the word "so", on the exhale, think the word "hum".

With your attention on what you hear, begin to feel your heart beating more strongly.

As you experience the beating of your heart, begin to experience gratitude.

The way you experience gratitude is to think of all the things, memories, and relationships in your life that you are grateful for.

Think of all the people whom you love and all the people who love you and all the people who share their love with you.

Gradually both the breath and the sound will become quieter and quieter, and eventually, the breath becomes so quiet that it almost seems to stop.

By quieting your breath, you quiet your mind. Time seems to stop, and you enter the field of pure consciousness, spirit.

In every tradition, mantras involve chanting to create special vibrations and sounds of the universe that created something from nothingness.

Mantra moves energy from the unmanifest into the manifest.

The sutra is a mantra that has meaning.

The mantra itself has no meaning. It is just a vibration, a sound. The word sutra is a Sanskrit word, related to the Latin noun Sutura, which is the base of the English word suture, meaning to join together by sewing.

A sutra is actually a stitch on the soul, and the stitch is one of intention.

Both mantras and sutras allow you to transcend to a deeper consciousness.

Therefore, you could use the "so-hum" mantra to transcend. Then you could use an actual word, a sutra, for a particular intention into your consciousness.

There are mantras and sutras that have been used for thousands of years. Even if the sounds are foreign to you and you don't understand their meaning, it does not diminish their effectiveness.

You do not have to understand the meanings of the sutras in order for them to work.

The soul will understand their meaning even if you do not.

Why do we use these ancient words as mantras and sutras instead of modern language? It is because of the potency.

Using newer mantras and sutras only makes the process of experiencing synchronicity more difficult.

There are many paths that will lead you home, the one that is familiar and that has been taken many times is the easier journey.

Similarly, mantras and sutras that have been used for thousands of years by millions of people over generations provide the easiest route to transcendence and spirit.

Every time a mantra or sutra is used, it helps increase the probability that a similar outcome will result from using the same mantra.

This means that the more a sutra is used, the greater the likelihood that its chosen intention will be fulfilled.

Therefore, it is better to use an old, well used sutra than a new sutra.

Try not to be put off by the use of Sanskrit but welcome the ancient words as allies in your search for the transcendence that leads to spirit.

Goddess

(Deity)

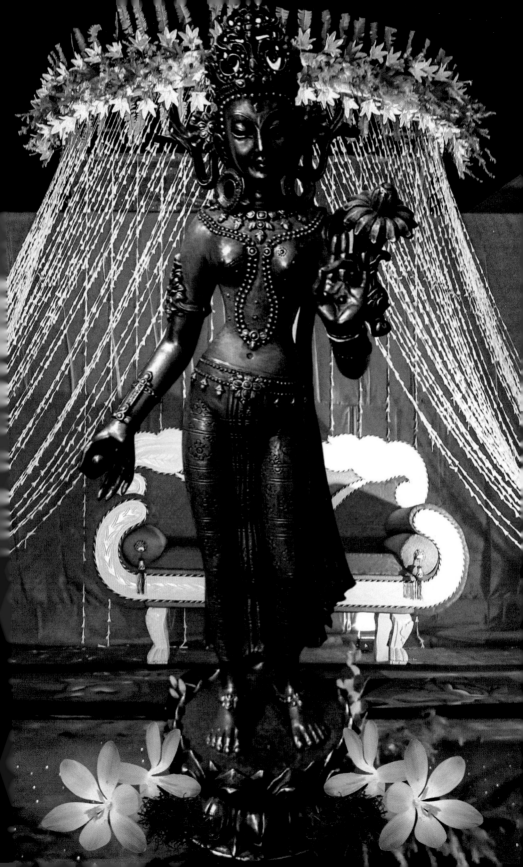

Who is Lakshmi?

There are seven auric fields that opens to different energy planes and energy bodies and also partners with a chakra, thus exchanging information between the worlds outside and inside of the body.

A chakra refers to energy points in your body. It is the point where the energetic and physical bodies meet.

The word chakra means "wheel" in Sanskrit and symbolises the flow of energy in our body. A chakra is a circular-shaped energy body that directs life energy for physical and spiritual well-being.

The body is a temple, and the chakras are switches in the body.

Kundalini Shakti and the divine grace and beauty of the mother can be awakened just by invoking the energies of the Chakras through mantra.

This is the essence of Sri Vidya.

Sri Vidya is the holiest, purest, and most powerful meditation of the universe.

It is the practice of Tantra that provides the framework for experiencing spiritual freedom and worldly pleasure.

Tantra originates in India and represents the sacred union of feminine and masculine energy dating back to the Indus Valley Civilisation (2000 BC) but scholars consider the main strains emerged between 300-400 AD.

It is the dance of the by-polar energy of Shiva and Shakti, the masculine and feminine archetypes, the sun and the moon, night and day, life, and death.

This duality is found in everything that exists in nature, it's a never-ending cycle that remains in balance.

A deep understanding of reality reveals that there is actually no duality, these two poles are two sides of the same coin.

Since everything has a divine nature, so do we.

Your life is very precious, mantras are about you and your deity (God /Goddess).

This deity is not someone else, it is your own soul.

We cannot see our soul, it is formless, that is why we give it a form.

The truth is the deity, and you are one.

The universe is exactly replicated in the human body.

Based on this idea, the creative force of the universe dwells in the letters of the alphabet, and in the nerve centres of the body as well, concentrating to develop the divine power within us.

The Tantra system closely follows Vedic injunctions. All forms of ceremonies of the present day are observed in accordance with tantras.

Let's meet the Sri behind Sri Vidya.

Sri is all aspects of the awakening of kundalini Shakti that leads to living a completely fulfilled, abundant, healthy, compassionate, beauty-filled, and gracious life.

Understanding Sri is understanding how to live fully and become a full Shakti.

Sri fills our hearts with divine bliss. Sri makes this life beautiful.

Maha Lakshmi represents the aspects of female cosmic energy, represents fertility, abundance, prosperity, riches, brilliance, and beauty.

Lakshmi is the most lustrous divine damsel endowed with unparalleled beauty, unearthly charm, and timeless youth, richly bejewelled and costumed, usually in red and possessed of the oceans of wealth.

Sri is Maha Lakshmi.

Sri is Tara, Durga, Kali, Saraswati, Guanyin, Kamla, and to them all we chant SHREEM.

The Maha Lakshmi Beej (seed) sound

SHREEM

SH - Auspicious, Grace, Beauty, Abundance - Maha Lakshmi

RA - The fire to activate - Durga/Kali

EEM - The river of consciousness from Shiva Shakti to the body and up again - Maha Saraswati.

SHREEM

We look for our voice to be sweeter, our heart to be more open and to be more creative and powerful, we open ourselves up to fearlessness. We give them all names, but we are chanting one sound.

SHREEM

Where we can open the door for grace to come into us and all the wonderful things to come into our life.

SHREEM

As above, so below and as below so above, all meeting at the heart.

There are teachings everywhere, look inward and ask yourself, why are you here?

Appreciate All!!

Find the gifts in your struggles. Forgive yourself and release yourself.

What you seek is seeking you. The universe is nothing but abundance.

SHREEM, SHREEM, SHREEM

There is one power in the universe, and I am a perfect manifestation of that power. As such I will that the boundaries of my aura shall be strong, beautiful, and healthy energy, safe within these boundaries, nothing can harm me, for I am filled with the strength of the God/Goddess. By my will, so mote it be and so it is.

Let the visual image of light shine bright within and around you and know that the protection and strength remain with you.

All teachings in Sri Vidya were given to Raja Choudhury by Guruji Amritananda of Devipuram, who in turn has shared the wisdom with me, so that I may now in turn, share that wisdom with you.

I am honoured and privileged.

So much gratitude and a great big thank you, Raja for being a part of my life and a part of this journey.

Mantras

Lakshmi

Maha Lakshmi

Om Shreem Hreem Shreem Kamle Kamlalaye Praseeda Praseeda

Shreem Hreem Shreem Om Maha Lakshmiye Namaha

Kamle Kamlalaye-She who comes out of the Red Lotuses, energies of the

moon and sun.

Praseeda Praseeda - to give and receive her grace.

Maha Lakshmiye - O Maha Lakshmi

Namaha - there is no me, just everything.

Meditation

Channelling the higher self

Quiet the mind, breathe deeply, focus inward and let go of worry.

White, cleansing light is all around you.

Your intention is to ask your higher self for assistance.

I invoke the I Am in me to connect to my higher self.

I invoke the I Am in me to send light energy to my body, healing my mind, heart, and soul/spirit.

I invoke the I Am in me to receive my highest and best insights.

Notice new insights that come to mind, trust your answers, have a feeling of rightness.

Ask yourself, how can everyone win?

Affirm that you have all the answers within and that you know what they all are already.

Picking up Stones and naming them.

Stones have an essence, there are many types, and each has a different story behind what went into forming each one.

They look different, behave different and weather differently.

The stones are alive.

When you want to cleanse yourself of emotions that are challenging, take a walk in nature, or by the ocean and look for stones that call out to you.

Select three stones that call out to you, the ones that feel good in your hands.

Name each stone by the label of whatever you are harbouring, names such as fear, guilt, shame, despair, frustration, and anger.

Carry these stones with you wherever you go.

Keep them in your pockets, alongside your nightstand and even bring them in the shower with you, when you bathe.

Develop a relationship with the stones.

When you have a rough day, lean on your stones.

Try to believe that they understand you, and that their job is to absorb the emotions you have named them.

The healing frequency of the minerals will act as an antidote to what ails you, whether physical, emotional, or spiritual.

If you lose a stone, it is not your fault. This is part of the experience.

You may replace them if you wish, or perhaps the emotion was ready to leave you.

When the time naturally comes that you feel the stones have done their job, carry them to a body of water and release them, and let the living water purify the venom they've drawn from you, and you will walk away purified, too.

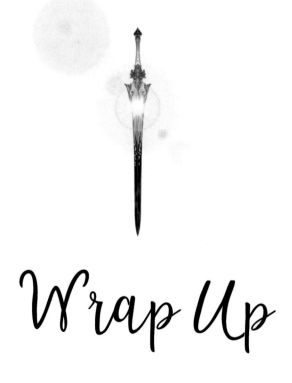

Wrap Up

The tiny seed knew that in order to grow it needed to be dropped in dirt, covered in darkness, and struggle to reach light.

Strong roots anchor the tree into the ground, providing everything it needs to thrive.

You too have physical and spiritual roots.

When your roots are strong, you most likely experience a sense of stability, connection, and ease because you are grounded.

What a powerful thing to be rooted and grounded in love, here on earth and connected to spirit above.

Love courses through you, giving you all you need for growth, healing and vitality.

Love is the constant that allows you to weather every season of your life.

You are transformed and re-created over and over again each year, blossoming into a newer, brighter version of yourself, recorded for all time on your soul.

You are here on earth to treasure each of life's moments and cherish those precious memories.

You are here to awaken your inner light and shine your light into the world.

Take a good look at your life and simplify anything that adds more stress.

Incorporate a nourishing diet, one that promotes a healthy body, mind, and soul, will help you refine your thoughts and weed out self-limiting thought patterns.

It is time to design your life, and that takes self-discipline. It takes care and thought.

Life runs on rhythms. Life needs different things at different times. When you are young you need adventure, when you are in middle age, you need stability and when you are old, you need rest.

Generalisations, but when we stay with the simple rhythms, generally we will be our happiest. It's a simple recipe.

Be simple, be rebellious, be powerful, be loving and joyous, be light.

Immerse yourself in things that feel good, appreciate being on the receiving end of things and savour your experiences.

It is important to carve out time for yourself and engage your senses. Reconnect back to mother nature and the heavens.

It is important to prioritize pleasure and intimacy for their own sake and turn them into a unique self-expression.

Simplify every aspect of your life, inner and outer. Your thoughts will become simple, even though you can still embrace the complex, your heart will be open and simple, even though it will be compassionate towards the difficulties of others.

In time, everyone will come to you because you have the one thing they seek, simplicity, it's just that simple.

You must clear away the weeds and add a rich fertilizer. The richer the soil, the more abundant your inner garden will become.

In order for this to happen you have to purify your life.

The universe wants to upgrade your life. You go through the breakdowns so that you can have breakthroughs.

In order to make a huge upgrade in your reality the endings are supposed to happen.

Every new beginning requires an ending.

Every day you get to choose the way your world looks, regardless of how you were raised or what you were taught to believe, you get to decide where your story goes from here.

Now is the time to immerse yourself in all things that support your life purpose.

You will feel a deep sense of satisfaction and relief when you have found your way, an inner knowing that the direction in which you are headed has aligned with what is intended.

When you connect to your body and truly listen to it and give it the nourishment that it truly desires, everything changes.

True miracles happen.

Make your well-being your priority on all levels and keep aligned to this truth.

Be guided by your inner stillness and let the universe help you upgrade your reality.

Be open to new opportunities, and possibilities.

Let the old go away gracefully.

Be resilient and open to the beautiful changes that await you.

You are never alone throughout the process, be gentle with yourself and know that you are exactly where you are meant to be, right here in this present moment, connected to everything there is and ever will be.

Let's rejoice at the coming of Universal Love into the world, let it pierce us to the core of our being, no one can escape the fiery rays of this love.

For wherever one hides, there you are.

Whoever you may be, there you are, beating in the heart of hearts.

Let's rejoice in the joy and laughter that follows unconditional love, open our hearts and minds to this vision of heaven as it dawns on earth.

There is beauty all around you and light finds you when you realize, you are part of that beauty and worth cherishing.

If we despise any, we journey to despise ourselves.

Look around and choose to see all as beautiful, it is your choice, what you choose.

Just know that it all begins and ends with each beautiful breath.

Let us take a moment of deep appreciation and gratitude to the creator for that which has been created.

Knowing that within our hearts we carry joy, peace, compassion, and love and so much more.

The beauty of this wisdom is ageless.

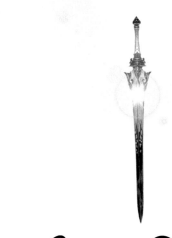

Next Step

ORGANISE YOUR
FREE DISCOVERY SESSION

A Free Discovery Session is a good place to start.
To look at your life through the lens of the 8 Seeds of Reverse Aging
to see where you need support and how we can help on the next step in your journey.

WITH

Wendy Jones

SIMPLY VISIT
WWW.AGELESS-WISDOM.COM
TO BOOK YOUR SESSION ONLINE

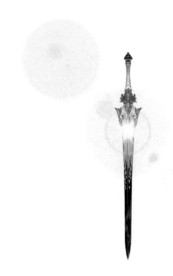

Offerings

BOOK | EBOOK
KEYNOTE SPEAKING

Events | Conferences | Summits | Webinars | Podcasts

Retreats | Workshops | Seminars

Transformational Coaching | Therapeutic Coaching

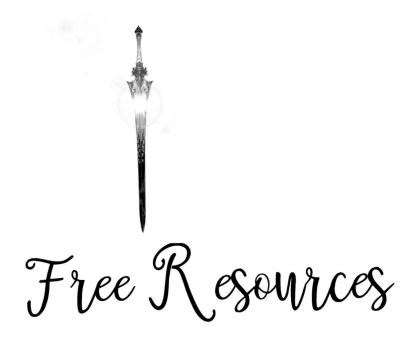

Free Resources

WWW.AGELESS-WISDOM.COM/RESOURCES

Testimonials

Once, during a ceremonial integration period, my dear Wendy came out with this little gem of word wisdom: 'smiles are for free!' I'd already known Wendy for several years and experienced her exuberance and playful soul, but to hear such a succinct clarification of how each of us could face The World and live youth-FULLY, set my brain-cogs a-whirling. Smiles ARE for free, and the bounty there from ripples out exponentially.

I'd first met Wendy during a vacation with friends to Virginia Beach. She was a friend of a friend, but immediately we clicked, and I knew from moment One that we were Kindred Spirits; Soul Sisters having known one another through time and time again. We talked, laughed, danced, played together, and cooked together. We left that vacation with a deep seeded understanding that we would always be in one another's life, that our paths were no longer parallel, but entwined from now on.

Since that weekend there have been many others when we have gathered to hold space, bask in Nature, play, dance, or just sit quietly. I have a degree of trust in Wendy that, for me and my history, can be difficult to place in "just anyone". On a spiritual and cellular level, I know I can ask her anything without fear of criticism or judgement of any kind. I can be my true unique self in her presence, and from observing others interacting with Wendy, I find the same to be true of them too. I sincerely believe anyone reading this book will put it down with that same feeling of trust and reception. Wendy is so relatable, and she reminds everyone she comes into contact with of their own inner child, and to realize their own innate ability to shed doubts and fears. Ultimately accepting Universal Love as our own Truth and Source.

I've seen Wendy during ceremonial settings, glide in like an Angel to the exact person in need of an assisting hand. No words were expressed, she simply sat by them, held them, or chanted over them. I've had her reach out to me when I've felt lonely, but not told anyone, and she'll have sent a text or maybe a package in the mail with a tender note.

Knowing and growing with Wendy these last few years, I've been blessed to witness her path towards healing unfold. I was an infant on my own healing path, able to ask her for guidance, or comfort, or techniques such as Sanskrit chanting or dietary hacks depending on my interests or needs. Her background in cosmetology often leads me to seek her advice on hair care or skin and beauty, but her knowledge and, yes, I'll just say it: Wisdom!, on so many subjects aligning mind/body/spirit has me diving into conversations with her that make me Think, and Feel, and Intuitively Know. Her passion, curiosity, and focused research means I can depend on her to have vetted out the distractions and get down to the nitty-gritty. We may not always 100% of the time come to the same conclusions, or agree on everything, but I can expand my perspective by asking myself questions such as: Why does Wendy feel that way about such-n-such? Is this thing I'm about to do (or take/try) something Wendy would have an alternative viewpoint on? How would Wendy handle this situation/personality/etc…?

She is to me a living, breathing embodiment of the Triple Goddess. All elements of Maiden/Mother/Crone shine through her to humbly show that we don't need all the walls, or veils, or distractions to be our True Selves. We just need to Smile.

I smile absolutely whenever I think of her. When a memory pops into my head, or I wonder what she's been doing, or my daughters and I moue (that's French for: to pout 😉) saying we really miss her and can't wait to see her... I can not help but smile that she's come into my life. Our lives.

So, I smile with her, and for her, and I send all the Free Smiles I can put into the Universe for YOU, dear reader, because of her.

Kristy Wasilewski | February 5, 2023

Wendy Jones is a dear friend, mentor, teacher, influencer & guide in the most subtle and brilliant ways. We've covered so many of life's "big topics", and I always walk away from the experience with greater grounding, self acceptance and a mood boost. What I love about Wendy's approach is her laughter, authenticity and non-judgment. It's as if Wendy knows we all show up doing the very best we know how to do, at any given moment, and from that perspective, we can release expectations and allow more open hearted healing to occur. However, my favorite quality of Wendy's is her reminder that this journey is meant to be fun, filled with love, yet FUN!

-Felicia Greenfield-Blau

Wendy came into my life during a time of midlife transition. She is an excellent listener, employing a grounding presence and empathy. She provided me with relatable spiritual guidance in my journey. Her sound and mantra healing created resonance for me and was an essential component in my awakening. Her spirit and gifts will be with me for a long time and for that I am grateful. – Shivad, Fairfax, VA

Hello, let me tell you a short story. Do you know Wendy? I do, she has been a friend of mine for about 3 years now. That of course is not a long time in the grand scheme of things, but time is relative so maybe I have known Wendy for 300 years. Either way, I would like to share some things about her. First, I shall mention a favorite author of mine. His name is Joseph Chilton Pearce and I have read his books many times. In one book of his he stresses, quite thoroughly, the importance of having in the flesh, real life guides or mentors. Role models. Well, I happen to agree with him. This is something many of us who grow up in modern society are missing from our lives. I think they used to call them elders. Where have all the elders gone? That's a song, right? Well, I have news for you, the elders are coming back around. Wendy, I think may even be one of them. Even if she is not an elder (she is!) she has most certainly been a role model for myself and for my daughters. She has often guided me in small ways as well. She was one of the first to impress upon me the concept of the inner child. It was a concept I had heard of a few times before, but it was a short conversation with Wendy, and I UNDERSTOOD what the whole thing was about. It's funny because I hadn't really thought about the inner child or that conversation for some time now but when Wendy asked me to write these words in support of her it came rushing back to mind. Probably a synchronicity because just the week before my wife picked up a book about inner bonding which discusses the inner child and other concepts related to that. I have been reading it and thinking on it and it explains a lot. There is a lot of discussion in the book about trust and how shame, blame, guilt, etc break the trust between an adult and a child. And I myself, independently of the book, have been meditating on the concept of trust and relationships for a few weeks now.

Over the course of these few weeks, I have been slowly analyzing how trust, or the lack thereof, has affected my personal relationships. Which begs the question: do I trust Wendy? Heavens yes!!!! Heavens YES, is the resounding answer. If we are all on a big ship (we are!) and only one person can steer at a time I would not hesitate to have Wendy take the wheel. I do not say this lightly. I am not much of a follower, and I have pretty high standards for a leader/elder, so it is no small thing, in my eyes, to say YES, we can trust Wendy to steer us to safe waters. I say us, because, I am taking this journey with you, the dear reader. I am going to be reading this book right along with you and I will be soaking up all the wisdom I can along the way.

David Wasilewski

If you would like an injection of joy.... Wendy's the real deal.

Lisa Jacenich

Wendy Jones is a powerhouse; intelligent, organized, insightful. She's a team player and a leader, skillful in group dynamics, and one on one. She has shared with me what she has learned in spirituality, health and fitness, providing easy to follow guidelines that have made my journey to greater wellbeing clearcut and manageable. She deals in facts, not fantasies, provides the evidence, not opinion. She does it in a way that is inspiring and exciting. I have known her for several years, and consider her a friend and mentor. She is always upbeat, authentic and truthful. I would love to work with her, knowing that she would always give her all to whatever endeavor, whatever enterprise. I can count on her to have my back. And I can count on her to tell me when I've gone off course. Wendy exudes confidence. She is a person I want in my closest circle, because I know I can count on her no matter what. 4m

James Jacenich

Why 8 Seeds?

The Number 8 resonates with authority, self-confidence, inner-strength, inner wisdom, and at the same time has love for humanity and a desire for peace.

Victory, prosperity and overcoming.

One of the most desired numbers. Number 8 is a source of power and strength.

The number 8 signifies balance. The vibrations of the number 8 are similar to the vibrations of the planet Earth.

The intensity and power of 8's energy can never be underestimated. 8 is also the lucky number of symmetry, which symbolizes order.

The vibration of 8 indicates that there is a need to look at situations in life from all angles before making any decisions.

8 is an even-numbered sign showing great balance and stability, selflessness, responsibility and resilience - in addition has no negative or opposite energy associated with it.

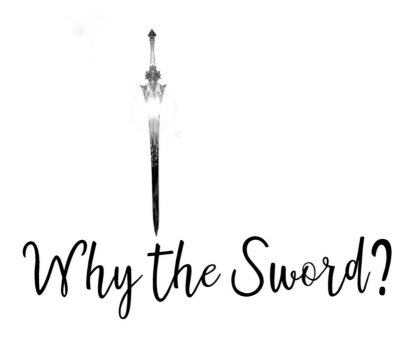

Why the Sword?

The sword symbolizes strength, power, dignity, leadership, light, courage, and vigilance.

It is an emblem of intelligence and, by extension, of the victory of spiritual knowledge, which opens the path to enlightenment.

The Vishnu Purana says that Nandaka, "the pure sword", represents jnana (knowledge), which is created from vidya (translated variously as wisdom, knowledge, science, learning, scholarship, philosophy), its sheath is avidya (ignorance or illusion).

The sword are used to represent a cutting of cords or energies that no longer serve you.

Archangel Michael calls us to Truth, Integrity and Power. He demands that we develop and rely upon our inner knowing and the spiritual worlds.

To develop this within us, he will strip away all that which belongs to the old, and anything that is 'no longer true' for us. Michael's energy is very powerful and unmistakenly fiery!

He uses his sword to cut and bless. Archangel Michael and his blue lightning Angels bring instant protection. Michael calls us to speak our truth and stand in our power as an IAMness.

Archangel Michael is very close in our consciousness at this time heralding the new age - an age of resurrection, of joy.

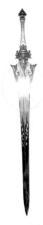

PRINT ON DEMAND

All titles by Wendy Jones are available at special quantity discounts for bulk purchases to be included for marketing, promotions, fundraisers and or education purposes.

You could also use them as a giveaway or as a gift with purchase for your valued clients or on the shelf in your library.

Contact wendy@ageless-wisdom.com to discuss how we can accommodate your needs.

Made in the USA
Columbia, SC
11 July 2023

20256538R00113